Cardiac arrhythmias

EXERCISES IN PATTERN INTERPRETATION

Cardiac arrhythmias

EXERCISES IN PATTERN INTERPRETATION

Mary H. Conover, R.N., B.S.

Instructor in Critical Care Nursing and Advanced Arrhythmia Workshops,
West Park and West Hills Hospitals, Canoga Park, Calif.;
formerly at California State University, Northridge,
and College of the Canyons, Valencia, Calif.

SECOND EDITION

with 256 ECG tracings

The C. V. Mosby Company

Saint Louis   1978

SECOND EDITION

Copyright © 1978 by The C. V. Mosby Company

Previous edition copyrighted 1974

Printed in the United States of America

Distributed in Great Britain by Henry Kimpton, London

The C. V. Mosby Company
11830 Westline Industrial Drive, St. Louis, Missouri 63141

Library of Congress Cataloging in Publication Data

Conover, Mary H
   Cardiac arrhythmias.

  Bibliography: p.
  Includes index.
  1. Arrhythmia. 2. Electrocardiography.
3. Arrhythmia—Nursing. I. Title. [DNLM:
1. Arrhythmia—Nursing texts. 2. Electrocardiography—Nursing texts. WY152.5 C753c]
RC685.A65C59 1978   616.1'28   77-24509
ISBN 0-8016-1024-9

CB/CB/CB 9 8 7 6 5 4 3 2 1

To

MY HUSBAND

whose patience, understanding, and encouragement have made my authorship possible,

MY CHILDREN

in gratitude to God, and

MY PARENTS

whose life and love continue to inspire me.

PREFACE

Cardiac Arrhythmias has been written in response to a need for practical experience in arrhythmia detection. Each chapter concentrates on one area of the heart or one division of electrocardiography and provides enough tracings to solidify the steps in arrhythmia detection.

New features of this second edition are as follows. Most of the first edition tracings have been replaced with new ones. Discussion has been expanded in each chapter regarding the fine points of arrhythmia diagnosis, the most current explanation of mechanism, and the physiology and pathophysiology of the structure under study. Two new chapters have been added. One is on laddergrams and gives you practice in the use of this valuable tool. The other is composed of test tracings taken from examinations I have given in the past to both basic and advanced groups. In this way you will have some idea of how successful your study program has been and what you would be expected to know about arrhythmias before working in a coronary care unit.

In the work space under each tracing you are prompted to make the step-by-step deductions that will lead to accurate conclusions in arrhythmia detection. If you sustain these deductive methods throughout the book, you will have established a habit, and you will seldom miss a diagnosis. Below the work section, the answer is supplied with an analysis of how you could have arrived at the correct diagnosis. ECG criteria, mechanisms, and hemodynamic consequences are discussed but not all at once under one arrhythmia. Instead, several examples of the same arrhythmia are offered. With each example new information is given so that you can slowly, step-by-step assimilate principles. By the end of each chapter you should have a good background in the electrophysiology, genesis, ECG characteristics, and clinical implications of a particular group of arrhythmias. Succeeding chapters will build on accumulated information.

To make the exercises more meaningful and to complete and round out your knowledge, I would advise you to read at least one of the references under each of the titles provided in the back of the book.

Most of the twelve leads seen in the chapter on myocardial infarction were given to me by Dr. Ara Tilkian. I am grateful to him for this and for making sure that there were no errors made in the interpretation of that chapter.

All of the other tracings in the book were faithfully collected by my students, the coronary care unit nurses of West Park Hospital, Canoga Park, California. I am grateful to them for their enthusiasm and help and to their unit director, Dr. Thomas Jacobson, for his encouragement and interest.

It is with great pleasure that I acknowledge Dr. Henry J. L. Marriott for his kindness to me and for the time he spent in reviewing the introduction to the chapter on aberrant ventricular conduction.

Mary H. Conover

CONTENTS

CHAPTER 1

ARRHYTHMIAS ORIGINATING IN THE SINUS NODE

Before attempting the pattern-reading exercises in this section, you should be familiar with the anatomy and physiology of the heart, cellular physiology, lead systems, normal electrical activation of the heart, and mechanism of arrhythmias originating in the sinus node.[1-4,20]

Basic to improving your diagnostic skills in arrhythmia interpretation is an understanding of the physiological role of the sinus node. The facility of applying this understanding to the interpretation of each arrhythmia may often greatly simplify the most complex-looking mechanism. Certainly in the face of an obscure mechanism, to discover that *at least* the sinus node is beating regularly unclutters the field (that is, eliminates any question of atrial ectopics).

FACTORS INFLUENCING INTRINSIC SINUS RATE

Under the control of the vagus nerves the sinus node responds to the physiological needs of the body. During sleep there is a normal slowing of the intrinsic sinus rate, and with exercise that rate increases to meet demand. Other factors also influence the functions of a normal sinus node. These include temperature, acetylcholine, catecholamines, atropine, and mechanical stretch (as would occur with right heart failure). Transient sinus nodal dysfunction may occur as a result of ischemia, increased intracranial pressure, and increased vagal tone. Overdrive suppression is demonstrated by the sinus node and by other cardiac pacemaker cells.[15-18] This is a phenomenon by which the intrinsic rate of pacemaker cells is depressed by an outside stimulus (for example, an atrial ectopic beat may depress the sinus rate momentarily).

P WAVE MORPHOLOGY

Throughout this chapter note the shape of the P waves. They all should be the same shape in the particular lead you are looking at. When the pacemaker focus is in the same place each beat, the vector will repeat identically each time, producing P waves that are all alike.

"WALKING OUT" A RHYTHM

At times the P waves will be perceived to be irregular when they are actually absolutely regular. This is especially true when the ventricular rhythm is irregular, and the sinus rhythm is not. You will very soon realize that it is best to "walk out" the sinus rhythm. This is done by finding two P waves in a row someplace in the tracing where you know that there is no chance that there could be a hidden P wave between the two apparent ones. Place a piece of paper under the P waves and mark them on the paper. Be sure that the mark is in the same place for each P wave. Then move your paper so that only one of the marks is on one of the P waves of the pair. Now, using the same two P waves, make another line under the P without the mark. Continue moving your paper and marking that same P wave until you have on the paper what you would expect of a normal sinus rhythm. Now compare the lines you have made with the P waves in the tracing. If every P wave comes out on a line and

1

if all of the P waves look alike, the patient has a sinus rhythm. This exercise will perhaps not be necessary in the beginning of this book. However, you will be surprised at what a help it will be later on when heart blocks are discussed. A caliper may also be used to walk out a rhythm.

P-R INTERVAL

The P-R interval is a measurement of atrioventricular conduction time. When the P-R interval is measured, you are evaluating the tracing for first-degree heart block or preexcitation syndrome (Wolff-Parkinson-White syndrome). Normally the P-R interval should not be more than 0.20 sec. or less than 0.12 sec. The term "P-R" is a little misleading because the measurement is from the beginning of the P wave to the beginning of the ventricular complex, which may be either a q or an r wave.

If you find that your interval measurements are consistently different from mine, perhaps you are not noticing the initial part of the QRS complex, in which case both your P-R and QRS measurements will be incorrect.

QRS DURATION

The QRS duration is a measurement of the time it takes for the ventricles to depolarize. The normal duration is usually given as 0.05 to 0.10 sec.

Q-T INTERVAL

The Q-T interval is a measure of the action potential from phase 0 to the end of phase 3. Primarily, it is equal to the refractory period of the heart. Because the length of the refractory period changes with heart rate, the Q-T interval changes also. It is, therefore, necessary to correct your measurement of this interval with heart rate. This is done by using the table provided in the appendix on p. 262. It is not as reliable a measurement as the preceding ones because of the technical difficulties in attaining accuracy.

The Q-T interval can be prolonged as a result of myocardial ischemia, quinidine, and hypocalcemia. It will be shortened with digitalis, propranolol, phenytoin, and hypercalcemia.

EXERCISE 1-1

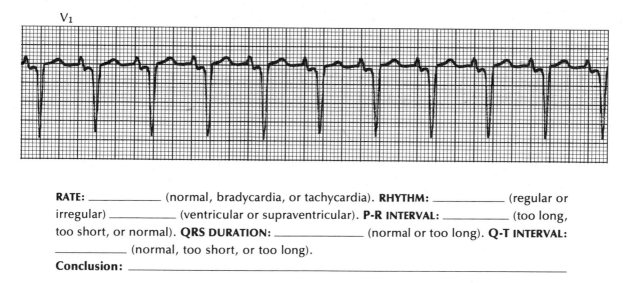

RATE: _____ (normal, bradycardia, or tachycardia). **RHYTHM:** _____ (regular or irregular) _____ (ventricular or supraventricular). **P-R INTERVAL:** _____ (too long, too short, or normal). **QRS DURATION:** _____ (normal or too long). **Q-T INTERVAL:** _____ (normal, too short, or too long).

Conclusion: _____

_____

ANALYSIS

RATE: 100/min. (normal). **RHYTHM:** regular and supraventricular. **P-R INTERVAL:** 0.14 sec. (normal). **QRS DURATION:** 0.09 sec. (normal). **Q-T INTERVAL:** 0.30 sec. (normal).

Conclusion: At a rate of 100 this rhythm is technically not a tachycardia. However, in the setting of the coronary care unit, *when the patient is at rest*, a rate of 100 should certainly cause you to search for a cause. Often a sinus tachycardia is the first sign of congestive heart failure. Certainly you should assess the patient, especially listening for a third heart sound and breath sounds. When cardiac output falls because of a failing left ventricle, the sinus node will increase its rate as a compensatory measure.

EXERCISE 1-2

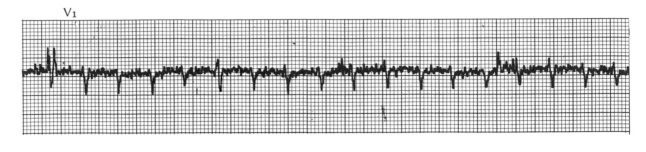

V₁

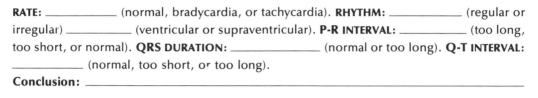

RATE: _____ (normal, bradycardia, or tachycardia). **RHYTHM:** _____ (regular or irregular) _____ (ventricular or supraventricular). **P-R INTERVAL:** _____ (too long, too short, or normal). **QRS DURATION:** _____ (normal or too long). **Q-T INTERVAL:** _____ (normal, too short, or too long).

Conclusion: _____

_____

ANALYSIS

RATE: 170-175/min. (tachycardia). **RHYTHM:** regular and supraventricular. **P-R INTERVAL:** impossible to determine. **QRS DURATION:** about 0.08 sec. (normal). **Q-T INTERVAL:** impossible to determine.

Conclusion: Apart from the fact that this is a supraventricular tachycardia, artifact makes it impossible to interpret any further. Artifact is anything on the ECG tracing that has not been produced by the heart, whether it is a pacemaker blip, hiccoughs, alternating current (AC) interference, or the tremor from another muscle other than the heart (somatic tremor). The artifact above is caused by a loose electrode. The disturbance should obviously be corrected so that a proper interpretation can be made of the ECG. This is especially true since the patient has a supraventricular tachycardia at a rate that threatens the cells of an already ischemic heart.

4

EXERCISE 1-3

V₁

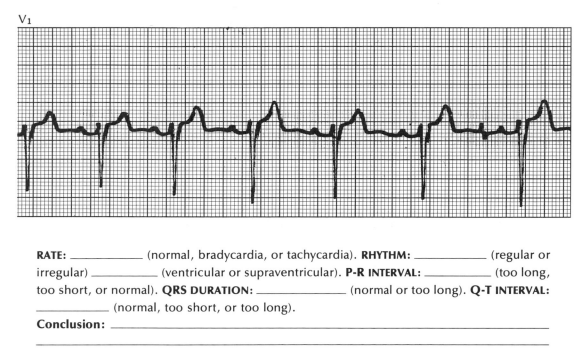

RATE: _____ (normal, bradycardia, or tachycardia). **RHYTHM:** _____ (regular or irregular) _____ (ventricular or supraventricular). **P-R INTERVAL:** _____ (too long, too short, or normal). **QRS DURATION:** _____ (normal or too long). **Q-T INTERVAL:** _____ (normal, too short, or too long).

Conclusion: _____

_____

ANALYSIS

RATE: 60-70/min. (normal). **RHYTHM:** irregular and supraventricular. **P-R INTERVAL:** 0.20 sec. (normal). **QRS DURATION:** 0.12 sec. (too long). **Q-T INTERVAL:** 0.38-0.40 sec. (normal).

Conclusion: This sinus arrhythmia has an artifact in it. Toward the end of the tracing there is a little blip that does not belong to, nor does it influence, the cardiac rhythm. You have probably also noticed the changing height of the ventricular complexes. This is the result of respirations and is termed "respiratory variations." It is normal and often seen. Sometimes these variations are so marked in lead II that they present a differential diagnosis with left anterior hemiblock (axis shift).

EXERCISE 1-4

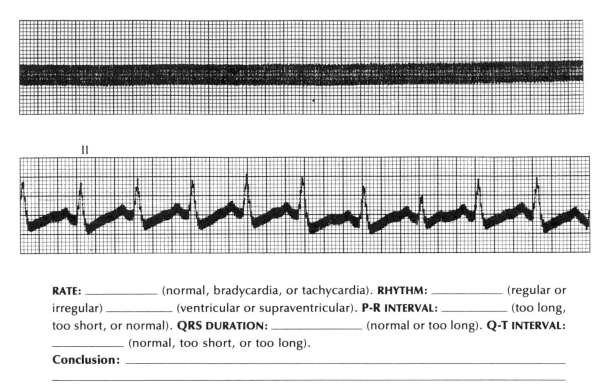

II

RATE: _____ (normal, bradycardia, or tachycardia). **RHYTHM:** _____ (regular or irregular) _____ (ventricular or supraventricular). **P-R INTERVAL:** _____ (too long, too short, or normal). **QRS DURATION:** _____ (normal or too long). **Q-T INTERVAL:** _____ (normal, too short, or too long).

Conclusion: _____

ANALYSIS

These two tracings are presented to illustrate the effect of AC on the graph, both without and with a concurrent ECG. The source of the interference should be identified and corrected. A 60-cycle AC artifact will always display an absolutely regular wave form that makes exactly 60 deflections/sec. This regular type of artifact is easily differentiated from the erratic artifact of patient movement (somatic tremor).

AC interference on the tracing can result from several causes and may or may not represent a hazard to the patient. The situation should be corrected at once.[1] If it is not due to a dry electrode pad or a defective patient cable, then defective electrical equipment in use on the patient should be suspected.

EXERCISE 1-5

II

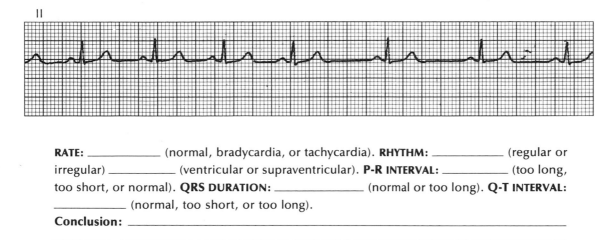

RATE: _____ (normal, bradycardia, or tachycardia). **RHYTHM:** _____ (regular or irregular) _____ (ventricular or supraventricular). **P-R INTERVAL:** _____ (too long, too short, or normal). **QRS DURATION:** _____ (normal or too long). **Q-T INTERVAL:** _____ (normal, too short, or too long).

Conclusion: _____

_____

ANALYSIS

RATE: approximately 65-70/min. (normal). RHYTHM: irregular and supraventricular. P-R INTERVAL: 0.12 sec. (normal). QRS DURATION: 0.08 sec. (normal). Q-T INTERVAL: 0.34 to 0.36 sec. (normal).

Conclusion: This is a sinus arrhythmia. The pacemaker is the sinus node, and conduction is normal. The rhythm is irregular in that it gradually slows down and then speeds up again. This is normal and is related to respiration. If the difference between the shortest R-R interval and the longest R-R interval is greater than 0.12 sec., the rhythm qualifies as a sinus arrhythmia. In this tracing that difference is 0.26 sec.

Note the difference between the first and the last Q-T interval. The Q-T accompanying the longer cycle is 0.02 sec. longer than that of the shorter cycle. This is because the refractory period changes with heart rate, becoming longer with bradycardia and shorter with tachycardia. The Q-T interval measures the action potential from phase 0 to the end of phase 3.

EXERCISE 1-6

V₁

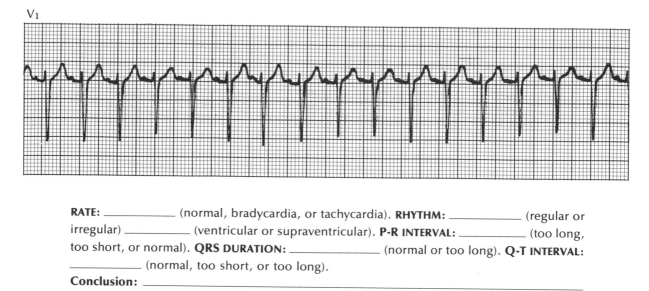

RATE: _____ (normal, bradycardia, or tachycardia). **RHYTHM:** _____ (regular or irregular) _____ (ventricular or supraventricular). **P-R INTERVAL:** _____ (too long, too short, or normal). **QRS DURATION:** _____ (normal or too long). **Q-T INTERVAL:** _____ (normal, too short, or too long).

Conclusion: _____

_____

ANALYSIS

RATE: 158/min. (tachycardia). **RHYTHM:** regular and supraventricular. **P-R INTERVAL:** 0.12 sec. (normal). **QRS DURATION:** 0.08 sec. (normal). **Q-T INTERVAL:** 0.26 sec. (normal).

Conclusion: This is a sinus tachycardia. A supraventricular tachycardia is certainly less serious than a ventricular tachycardia. However, it has been shown in animals and in man that atrial pacing rates of greater than 120-140/min. will cause a significant decrease in coronary arterial blood flow.[20-22] If this rate is allowed to continue in patients with acute myocardial infarction, a profound detriment in coronary perfusion may result. This in turn would aggravate ischemia, allowing the ventricles to become more vulnerable to ventricular fibrillation and cardiac arrest.

As stated in exercise 1-1, sinus tachycardia may be the first sign of congestive heart failure. You should certainly question the need for the sinus node to beat that fast when the patient is at rest. Sinus tachycardia is not treated. It is necessary to determine the cause and then to initiate appropriate measures.

EXERCISE 1-7

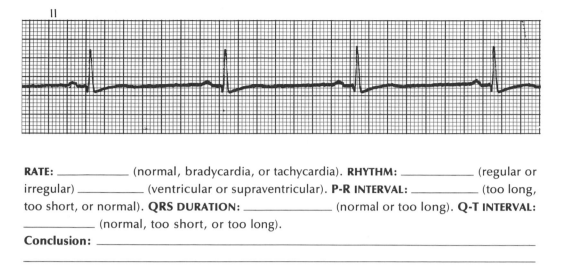

RATE: _____ (normal, bradycardia, or tachycardia). **RHYTHM:** _____ (regular or irregular) _____ (ventricular or supraventricular). **P-R INTERVAL:** _____ (too long, too short, or normal). **QRS DURATION:** _____ (normal or too long). **Q-T INTERVAL:** _____ (normal, too short, or too long).

Conclusion: _____

_____

ANALYSIS

RATE: 40-42/min. (bradycardia). RHYTHM: regular and supraventricular. P-R INTERVAL: 0.20 sec. (normal). QRS DURATION: 0.08 sec. (normal). Q-T INTERVAL: 0.52 sec. (too long).

Conclusion: This is a sinus bradycardia. The term "sinus" indicates that the pacemaker is the sinus node. The term "bradycardia" is used when the heart rate is below 60 beats/min. The P-R interval is normal, which rules out first-degree heart block. A normal QRS duration indicates normal intraventricular conduction time. In this case the Q-T interval is prolonged, indicating a lengthening of the refractory period. Myocardial ischemia, quinidine, and hypocalcemia are all causes of a prolonged Q-T interval. Hypokalemia will cause an additional hump (U wave) in the ECG after the T wave. This may appear to lengthen the Q-T interval (see figure on p. 14).

The clinical significance and treatment of sinus bradycardia in acute myocardial infarction has been a point of much controversy since 1972[24-39] when it was shown that serious ventricular dysrhythmias may result after the administration of atropine to patients with acute myocardial infarction and sinus bradycardia.[33,36] At present some observers feel that atropine should not be administered to patients with sinus bradycardia without ventricular irritability, hypotension, or evidence of pump failure, since these patients usually have a benign clinical course. However, it is further stated that when sinus bradycardia is complicated by hypotension, atropine is the drug of choice and that this drug can be used safely in patients with acute myocardial infarction as long as proper attention is paid to the dosage and the setting is that of a coronary care unit.[37]

EXERCISE 1-8

V₁

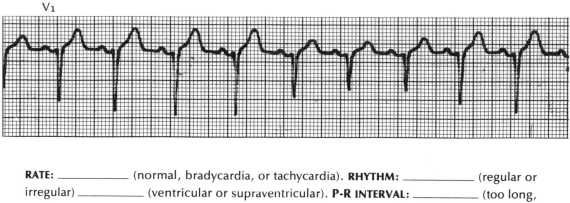

RATE: _____ (normal, bradycardia, or tachycardia). **RHYTHM:** _____ (regular or irregular) _____ (ventricular or supraventricular). **P-R INTERVAL:** _____ (too long, too short, or normal). **QRS DURATION:** _____ (normal or too long). **Q-T INTERVAL:** _____ (normal, too short, or too long).
Conclusion: _____
_____

ANALYSIS

RATE: 94-100/min. (normal) **RHYTHM:** regular and supraventricular. **P-R INTERVAL:** 0.14 sec. (normal). **QRS DURATION:** 0.08 sec. (normal).

Conclusion: This is a normal sinus rhythm. The rhythmically changing height of the S waves is the result of respirations (respiratory variations). With deep inspiration the heart position becomes more vertical, and with deep expiration it becomes more horizontal. The rotation of the heart is also affected; it rotates more clockwise during inspiration and counterclockwise during expiration.

EXERCISE 1-9

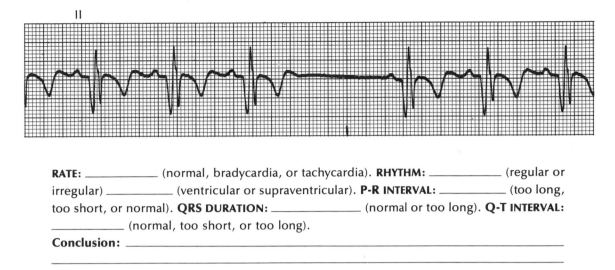

RATE: _____ (normal, bradycardia, or tachycardia). **RHYTHM:** _____ (regular or irregular) _____ (ventricular or supraventricular). **P-R INTERVAL:** _____ (too long, too short, or normal). **QRS DURATION:** _____ (normal or too long). **Q-T INTERVAL:** _____ (normal, too short, or too long).

Conclusion: _____

_____

ANALYSIS

RATE: approximately 70/min. (normal). RHYTHM: irregular and supraventricular. P-R INTERVAL: 0.18 sec. (normal). QRS DURATION: 0.14 sec. (too long). Q-T INTERVAL: 0.46 sec. (too long).

Conclusion: This is probably a sinus exit block or sinus arrest. Arrest and exit block of the sinus node cannot always be distinguished from each other in the ECG. The mechanism of sinus arrest is that of depression of impulse formation, whereas the mechanism of sinus exit block is that of depression of impulse conduction. In the above tracing one or the other has occurred spontaneously during a sinus rhythm.

When the diagnosis of sinus exit block or sinus arrest is made, there is a differential diagnosis. When unexpected pauses occur in the ECG, the *usual* cause is a nonconducted premature atrial contraction (PAC). Sinus arrest is far less common. This differential diagnosis is discussed in more detail in Chapter 2.

EXERCISE 1-10

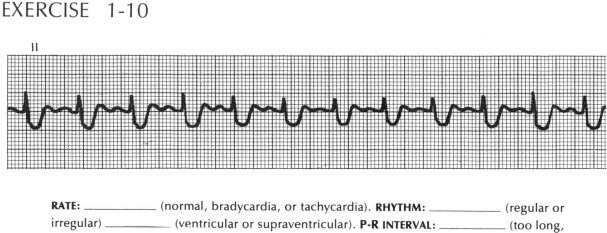

II

RATE: _____ (normal, bradycardia, or tachycardia). **RHYTHM:** _____ (regular or irregular) _____ (ventricular or supraventricular). **P-R INTERVAL:** _____ (too long, too short, or normal). **QRS DURATION:** _____ (normal or too long). **Q-T INTERVAL:** _____ (normal, too short, or too long).

Conclusion: _____

_____

ANALYSIS

RATE: 110-112/min. (tachycardia). RHYTHM: regular and supraventricular. P-R IN-TERVAL: 0.20 sec. (normal). QRS DURATION: 0.08 sec. (normal). Q-T INTERVAL: 0.32 sec. (normal).

Conclusion: This is a sinus tachycardia. Notice the scooped, pulled-down look of the S-T segment, a typical digitalis effect. Myocardial ischemia will also cause the S-T segment to be depressed. However, in the case of ischemia the Q-T interval would be prolonged, whereas digitalis causes a shortening. This is a helpful point to remember in the differential diagnosis of S-T segment depression.

The clinical implications of sinus tachycardia have already been discussed in exercises 1-1 and 1-6.

EXERCISE 1-11

V₁

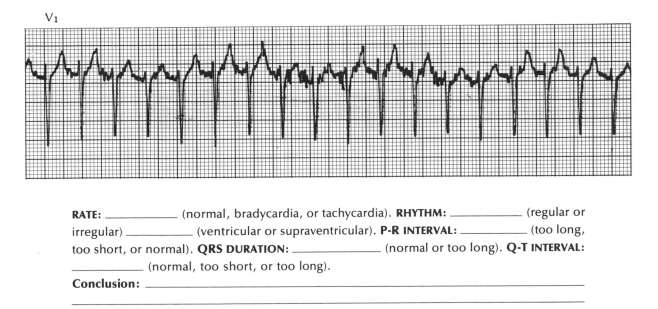

RATE: _____ (normal, bradycardia, or tachycardia). **RHYTHM:** _____ (regular or irregular) _____ (ventricular or supraventricular). **P-R INTERVAL:** _____ (too long, too short, or normal). **QRS DURATION:** _____ (normal or too long). **Q-T INTERVAL:** _____ (normal, too short, or too long).

Conclusion: _____

_____

ANALYSIS

RATE: 175/min. (tachycardia). RHYTHM: regular and supraventricular. P-R INTERVAL: impossible to determine. QRS DURATION: 0.08 sec. (normal). Q-T INTERVAL: impossible to determine.

Conclusion: This is a supraventricular tachycardia. Somatic tremor makes any further evaluation of the tracing impossible. Notice the difference between the irregular, erratic artifact of this muscle tremor and the absolute even regularity of AC interference (see figure on p. 6).

EXERCISE 1-12

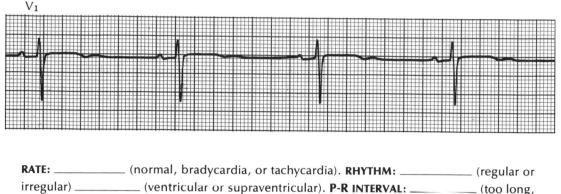

V₁

RATE: _____ (normal, bradycardia, or tachycardia). **RHYTHM:** _____ (regular or irregular) _____ (ventricular or supraventricular). **P-R INTERVAL:** _____ (too long, too short, or normal). **QRS DURATION:** _____ (normal or too long). **Q-T INTERVAL:** _____ (normal, too short, or too long).

Conclusion: _____

_____

ANALYSIS

RATE: 40/min. (bradycardia). **RHYTHM:** supraventricular and irregular. **P-R INTERVAL:** 0.18 sec. (normal). **QRS DURATION:** 0.08 sec. (normal). **Q-T INTERVAL:** 0.52 sec. (too long).

Conclusion: This is a sinus arrhythmia and sinus bradycardia. A U wave is easily seen in this tracing. It is the extra little hump after the T wave. These are seen in normal people and become prominent in hypokalemia. The ECG is a very sensitive indicator of the ratio of intracellular to extracellular potassium and shows signs of hypokalemia even when the serum potassium level is still within normal limits.

EXERCISE 1-13

II

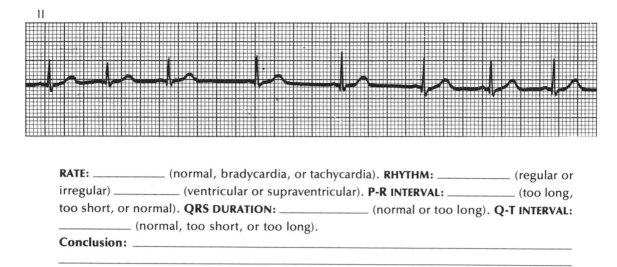

RATE: _____ (normal, bradycardia, or tachycardia). **RHYTHM:** _____ (regular or irregular) _____ (ventricular or supraventricular). **P-R INTERVAL:** _____ (too long, too short, or normal). **QRS DURATION:** _____ (normal or too long). **Q-T INTERVAL:** _____ (normal, too short, or too long).

Conclusion: _____

_____

ANALYSIS

RATE: approximately 85/min. (normal). RHYTHM: irregular and supraventricular. P-R INTERVAL: 0.12 sec. (normal). QRS DURATION: 0.08 sec. (normal). Q-T INTERVAL: 0.32 sec. (normal).

Conclusion: Since there is a difference of 0.32 sec. between the shortest and the longest cycle, this qualifies as a sinus arrhythmia. The tracing was taken from a healthy 4-year-old boy, and this particular arrhythmia is almost always present in well children. The person who is accustomed to looking at the adult ECG is very surprised to see such a degree of sinus arrhythmia so consistently in the child.

EXERCISE 1-14

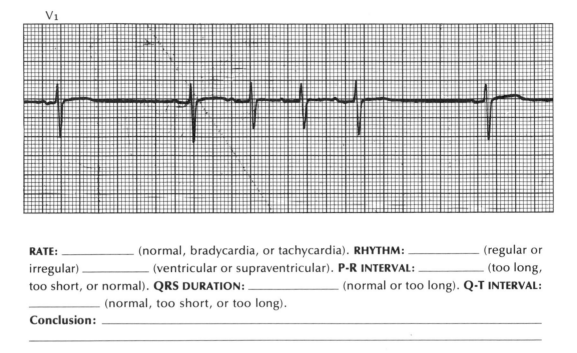

V₁

RATE: _____ (normal, bradycardia, or tachycardia). **RHYTHM:** _____ (regular or irregular) _____ (ventricular or supraventricular). **P-R INTERVAL:** _____ (too long, too short, or normal). **QRS DURATION:** _____ (normal or too long). **Q-T INTERVAL:** _____ (normal, too short, or too long).

Conclusion: _____

_____

ANALYSIS

RATE: Bradycardia-tachycardia. RHYTHM: irregular and supraventricular. **P-R INTER-VAL:** 0.16-0.22 sec. (too long, varies). **QRS DURATION:** 0.08 sec. (normal). **Q-T INTERVAL:** varies.

Conclusion: This tracing is from an adult and represents sick sinus syndrome, which manifests itself by alternating tachycardia and bradycardia and results in Adams-Stokes syndrome. This condition is often refractory to drugs and may require a pacemaker.[5-14]

CHAPTER 2
ATRIAL ECTOPICS

In this chapter you will learn to become more discerning in your evaluation of P waves and supraventricular rhythms. In the previous chapter the sinus rhythm has been noted in all of its variants. This search for the sinus rhythm should continue to be habitual. Remember that if all P waves emanate from the sinus node, they all will be the same shape in a particular lead. An ectopic P wave, which is called P' (prime), is usually of noticeably different morphology.

Since ventricular ectopics have not yet been introduced, all of the rhythms in this chapter are supraventricular (originate above the branching portion of the bundle of His).

You are also asked to note whether or not the rhythm is regular. So far we have dealt with only two causes of an irregular rhythm. They are sinus arrhythmia and sinus exit block. From now on you will become familiar with other causes of irregular rhythms: namely, premature atrial contractions (PACs), paroxysmal atrial or supraventricular tachycardia (PAT), chaotic atrial tachycardia (multifocal PACs), atrial flutter with variable A-V conduction, and atrial fibrillation. Sometimes the rhythm is regular even in the presence of an atrial ectopic arrhythmia, as in a sustained atrial tachycardia, atrial flutter with a consistent conduction ratio, and atrial fibrillation with complete heart block.

PACs are the result of enhanced automaticity, which may in turn be the result of any one of a number of causes, such as hypoxia, stretch of the conductive fibers, hypokalemia, hypocalcemia, heat, trauma, hypercapnia, catecholamines, and digitalis excess.

A single PAC can trigger atrial tachyarrhythmias, such as PAT, atrial flutter, and atrial fibrillation. Many investigators feel that such arrhythmias are supported by a reentry mechanism,[49-58] or, less commonly, are the result of repeated firing of a single focus. I refer you to the textbooks and periodicals for a more complete background in this subject.[1-4] Briefly, enhanced automaticity occurs when a group of myocardial cells develops the capacity to fire at an accelerated rate. Reentry occurs when impulses encounter a path of slow conduction coupled with one-way block.[50] Because it takes so long for the impulse to traverse the area of slow conduction, by the time it emerges the normal cardiac tissue is nonrefractory. The impulse can then reenter the nonrefractory tissue, and recapture takes place. If this circuit is sustained, a tachyarrhythmia results. Such an arrhythmia is easily interrupted by a well-timed electrical stimulus[49] or a lengthening of the refractory period in one of the pathways, both of which will break a link in the circuit. A single PAC can cause dissociation within the A-V node, placing one side of the node out of phase with the other so that the impulse goes round and round, capturing the ventricles each time (paroxysmal supraventricular, A-V nodal, junctional, or reciprocating tachycardia are all acceptable terms). A vagal maneuver may interrupt the circuit and terminate the tachycardia because such a maneuver lengthens the A-V nodal refractory period.

A PAC occurring during the relative refractory period of the atria may cause such a reentry circuit within the atrial specialized conductive system (internodal and interatrial tracts), resulting in atrial flutter.[58]

Reentry has also been reported to occur within the sinus node, resulting in atrial tachyarrhythmias (PAT).[51,52,54-58]

EXERCISE 2-1

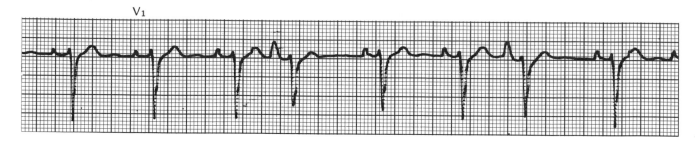

V₁

RATE: _____ (normal, bradycardia, or tachycardia). **RHYTHM:** _____ (regular or irregular) _____ (ventricular or supraventricular). **P-R INTERVAL:** _____ (too long, too short, or normal) _____ (absent P waves). **QRS DURATION:** _____ (normal or too long). **Q-T INTERVAL:** _____ (normal, too long, or too short). **P' WAVES:** _____ (present or absent).

Conclusion: _____

_____

ANALYSIS

RATE: 70/min. (normal). **RHYTHM:** irregular and supraventricular. **P-R INTERVAL:** 0.16 sec. (normal). **QRS DURATION:** 0.10 sec. (normal). **Q-T INTERVAL:** 0.35 sec. (normal). **P' WAVES:** present.

Conclusion: There are two PACs in this tracing (fourth and seventh beats). I hardly need to point them out since they are so huge compared with the sinus P waves and since they cause an irregularity in the rhythm because they are premature.

Start from the first P wave in the tracing and walk out the P-P intervals. You will find that the ectopic atrial beat causes the sinus node to reset itself, and the sinus P wave following the PAC comes earlier than it would have if the rhythm had not been interrupted. This is called a less than full compensatory pause, a certain sign of premature atrial depolarization. When such an event is less obvious, this is a helpful clue. Sometimes a PAC will have the opposite effect and will suppress the rate of the sinus node (overdrive suppression).[15-19] This phenomenon is illustrated on p. 22.

EXERCISE 2-2

II

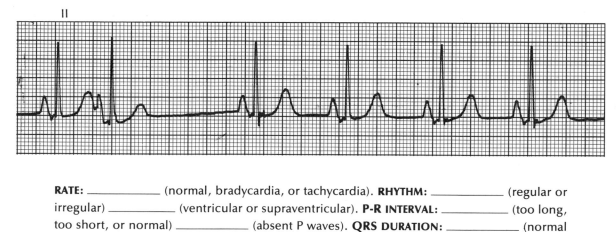

RATE: _____ (normal, bradycardia, or tachycardia). **RHYTHM:** _____ (regular or irregular) _____ (ventricular or supraventricular). **P-R INTERVAL:** _____ (too long, too short, or normal) _____ (absent P waves). **QRS DURATION:** _____ (normal or too long). **Q-T INTERVAL:** _____ (normal, too long, or too short). **P' WAVES:** _____ (present or absent).

Conclusion: _____

_____

ANALYSIS

RATE: 62/min. (normal). **RHYTHM:** irregular and supraventricular. **P-R INTERVAL:** 0.16 sec. (normal). **QRS DURATION:** 0.08 sec. (normal). **Q-T INTERVAL:** 0.42 sec. (normal). **P' WAVES:** present.

Conclusion: Here again a PAC causes an irregularity in the underlying sinus rhythm. The P' wave in this case is really close to the preceding T wave. Sometimes a P' wave that is this premature will not conduct at all because of the refractoriness of the ventricles or may be conducted abnormally for the same reason.

In this tracing we have another opportunity to notice how heart rate will change the action potential duration. The Q-T interval after the long pause is 0.06 sec. longer than the others.

In the setting of the coronary care unit the cause of frequent PACs should be investigated. They may be one of the first signs of congestive heart failure, since increased left ventricular pressure would be reflected back to the atria, causing stretch of the atrial conductive fibers and ectopic beats. Digitalis toxicity is also a consideration, as is hypoxia and acid-base imbalance.

EXERCISE 2-3

V₁

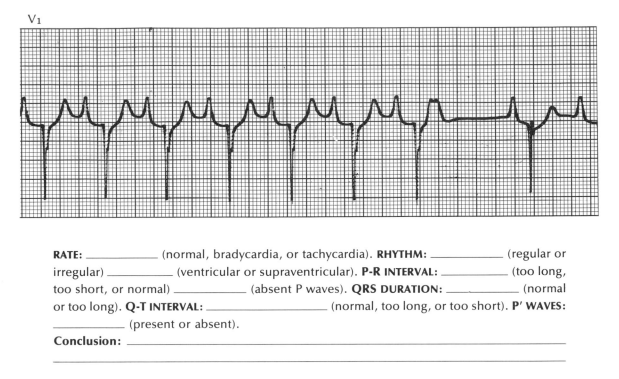

RATE: _____ (normal, bradycardia, or tachycardia). **RHYTHM:** _____ (regular or irregular) _____ (ventricular or supraventricular). **P-R INTERVAL:** _____ (too long, too short, or normal) _____ (absent P waves). **QRS DURATION:** _____ (normal or too long). **Q-T INTERVAL:** _____ (normal, too long, or too short). **P′ WAVES:** _____ (present or absent).

Conclusion: _____

ANALYSIS

RATE: 85-90/min. (normal). RHYTHM: irregular and supraventricular. P-R INTERVAL: 0.22 sec. (too long). QRS DURATION: 0.08 sec. (normal). Q-T INTERVAL: 0.32 sec. (normal). P′ WAVES: present.

Conclusion: Here is the great imitator, the nonconducted PAC. This arrhythmia is commonly incorrectly called sinus exit block or sinus arrest. Whenever you encounter an unexpected pause, remember that the nonconducted P′ is far more common than sinus exit block. Carefully examine the T wave preceding the pause and compare it with the other T waves in the tracing. They should all be the same shape. In this particular tracing the T wave before the pause has what appears to be an elevated S-T segment. If you compare this T wave with the others, you will notice that the elevation is caused by a hidden P′ wave.

There are two other features in this tracing that warrant your attention: first-degree heart block (long P-R interval) and junctional escape beat. The heart block is discussed in detail on p. 118. You would have been unaware of the junctional escape beat unless you are very discerning. Notice the following: (1) The P-R interval after the pause is shorter than the others because the latent pacemaker in the A-V junction fired and captured the ventricles before the sinus beat had a chance to do so; and (2) the ventricular complex after the pause is slightly different from the others. The latter is a very helpful sign in locating the junctional escape beats. The slight aberrancy occurs because sometimes the location of the junctional escape focus is a little offset within the A-V junction, causing the resultant ventricular complex to be ever so slightly aberrant.[58,59]

EXERCISE 2-4

V₁

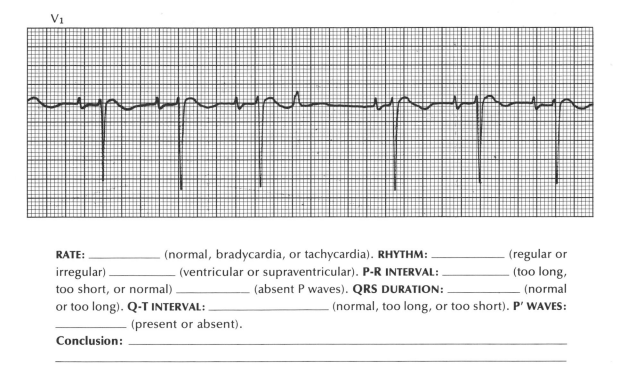

RATE: _____ (normal, bradycardia, or tachycardia). **RHYTHM:** _____ (regular or irregular) _____ (ventricular or supraventricular). **P-R INTERVAL:** _____ (too long, too short, or normal) _____ (absent P waves). **QRS DURATION:** _____ (normal or too long). **Q-T INTERVAL:** _____ (normal, too long, or too short). **P′ WAVES:** _____ (present or absent).

Conclusion: _____

_____

ANALYSIS

RATE: 72/min. (normal). RHYTHM: irregular and supraventricular. P-R INTERVAL: 0.22 sec. (too long). QRS DURATION: 0.09 sec. (normal). Q-T INTERVAL: 0.40 sec. (too long). P′ WAVES: present.

Conclusion: This tracing has some of the same features as the last. Did you pick them out? There is a nonconducted PAC, first-degree heart block, and junctional escape. The P′ wave is very obvious before the pause. First-degree heart block is determined because the P-R interval exceeds 0.20 sec. The junctional escape beat is noticed because the P-R interval following the pause is shorter than the others. In this case the junctional escape complex is exactly the same morphology as the sinus-conducted ones.

EXERCISE 2-5

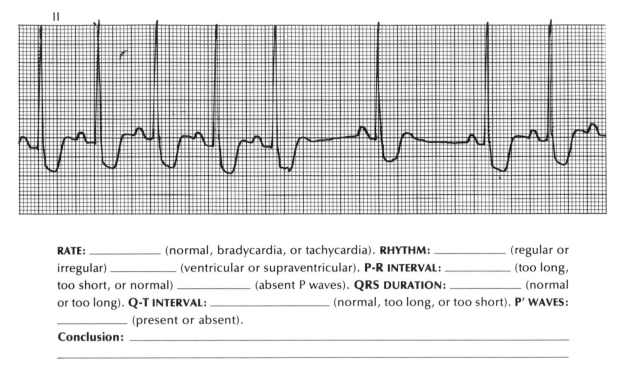

RATE: _____ (normal, bradycardia, or tachycardia). **RHYTHM:** _____ (regular or irregular) _____ (ventricular or supraventricular). **P-R INTERVAL:** _____ (too long, too short, or normal) _____ (absent P waves). **QRS DURATION:** _____ (normal or too long). **Q-T INTERVAL:** _____ (normal, too long, or too short). **P' WAVES:** _____ (present or absent).

Conclusion: _____

_____

ANALYSIS

RATE: approximately 80/min. (normal). **RHYTHM:** irregular and supraventricular. **P-R INTERVAL:** 0.19 sec. (normal). **QRS DURATION:** 0.08 sec. (normal). **Q-T INTERVAL:** 0.35 sec. (normal). **P' WAVES:** present.

Conclusion: There are two nonconducted PACs in this tracing. When you encounter an unexpected pause, this should be the first thing you think of. If you compare the T waves before the pause with the others, you can easily see the distortion caused by the hidden P' waves. Remember that all of the T waves should be the same shape.

Apart from distorting the T waves, the hidden P' waves manifest their presence in another way. Notice that the sinus rhythm after the last pause begins somewhat slower than the sinus rhythm preceding the pauses. This phenomenon is called overdrive suppression. It is a property of all pacemaker cells and means that the inherent rate of a pacemaker cell may be suppressed when that cell is stimulated from another source. For example, when the sinus node cells are stimulated by an ectopic focus, often one or two cycles occur before the sinus rate is back to what it was before the intrusion.[15-19]

Although somatic tremor distorts some of the tracing in the figure at the top of p. 23, it is evident that bigeminal nonconducted PACs simulate a sudden onset of sinus bradycardia. Because the treatment for sinus bradycardia and PACs is so completely different, it is important to make a differential diagnosis. The first PAC occurs after the second beat and is normally conducted. There is a nonconducted P' wave in the fourth T wave and in every T wave following.

If you remember the normal physiology of the sinus node and remember to compare T waves, the P' waves will be easily detected. The healthy sinus node does not suddenly jump into a sinus bradycardia or a sinus tachycardia. These arrhythmias ensue gradually in response to lessened or quickened body needs. The nonconducted PAC is more common than the condition it mimics, namely, sinus exit block.

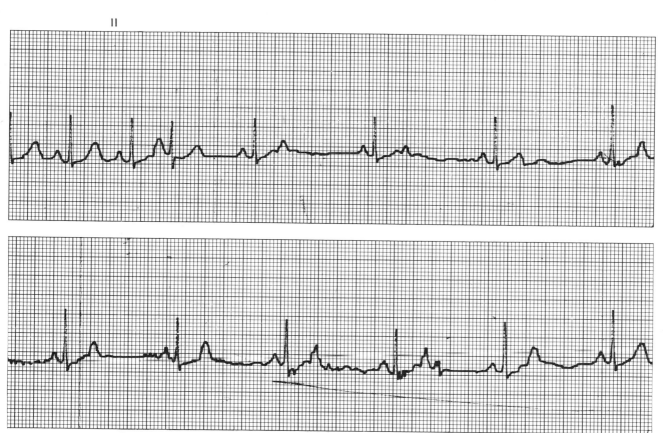

II

Continuous tracings. Bigeminal nonconducted PACs simulate sinus bradycardia.

The figure below is a sinus exit block. Notice that there are unexpected pauses, as in the previous tracings. However, on close examination, you cannot see any sign of distortion of the T wave before the pause. This, then, qualifies as a sinus exit block.

MCL₁

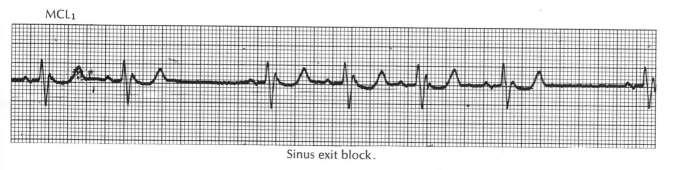

Sinus exit block.

EXERCISE 2-6

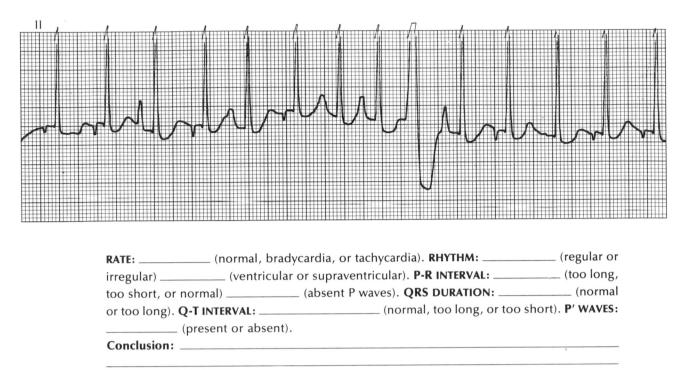

RATE: _____ (normal, bradycardia, or tachycardia). **RHYTHM:** _____ (regular or irregular) _____ (ventricular or supraventricular). **P-R INTERVAL:** _____ (too long, too short, or normal) _____ (absent P waves). **QRS DURATION:** _____ (normal or too long). **Q-T INTERVAL:** _____ (normal, too long, or too short). **P' WAVES:** _____ (present or absent).

Conclusion: _____

ANALYSIS

RATE: 115-160/min. (tachycardia). RHYTHM: irregular and supraventricular. P-R INTERVAL: absent P waves. QRS DURATION: 0.08 sec. (normal). Q-T INTERVAL: difficult to determine. P' WAVES: present.

Conclusion: In this tracing there are multifocal PACs, sometimes called chaotic atrial tachycardia. This arrhythmia is the one most commonly seen during acute respiratory failure.[4]

At least four different P' wave shapes can be seen throughout the strip. The first three P' waves are all different in morphology from each other and the third P' wave from the end is different still. These differences indicate that many ectopic foci are assuming pacemaker function in the atria.

There is one very broad ectopic looking ventricular complex in the tracing. This is discussed in Chapter 4.

EXERCISE 2-7

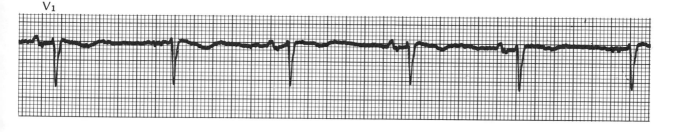

V₁

RATE: _____ (normal, bradycardia, or tachycardia). **RHYTHM:** _____ (regular or irregular) _____ (ventricular or supraventricular). **P-R INTERVAL:** _____ (too long, too short, or normal) _____ (absent P waves). **QRS DURATION:** _____ (normal or too long). **Q-T INTERVAL:** _____ (normal, too long, or too short). **P′ WAVES:** _____ (present or absent).

Conclusion: _____

_____

ANALYSIS

RATE: 48-50/min. (bradycardia). RHYTHM: regular and supraventricular. P-R INTERVAL: 0.20 sec. (normal). QRS DURATION: 0.09 sec. (normal). Q-T INTERVAL: 0.48 sec. P′ WAVES: present.

Conclusion: The atrial ectopic beats in this tracing are not premature. They are escape beats that occur because of sinus slowing. They are also fusion beats, firing at the same time as the sinus node. The two vectors, the one from the sinus node and the one from the ectopic focus, collide within the atria. Because the two forces are opposing each other, they cancel each other out, and the resultant P′ wave is isoelectric.

The patient's hemodynamic state does not change because of these escape atrial ectopics. It is a normal phenomenon that occurs when the sinus node is beating too slowly. After each heartbeat all of the pacemaker cells in the heart (sinus node and atrial and ventricular conductive system) begin to slowly depolarize in order to reach threshold and fire. The sinus node cells are normally the quickest at this. However, if they fail to fire on time, the latent pacemaker cells will continue to slowly depolarize. If threshold is reached before the sinus node discharges, these latent pacemaker cells will pace the heart for that beat. Such a beat is called an escape beat, either atrial, junctional, or ventricular, depending on its origin.

EXERCISE 2-8

II

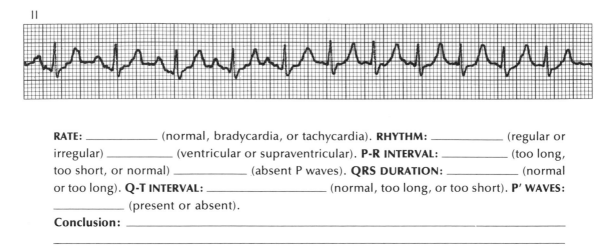

RATE: _____ (normal, bradycardia, or tachycardia). **RHYTHM:** _____ (regular or irregular) _____ (ventricular or supraventricular). **P-R INTERVAL:** _____ (too long, too short, or normal) _____ (absent P waves). **QRS DURATION:** _____ (normal or too long). **Q-T INTERVAL:** _____ (normal, too long, or too short). **P' WAVES:** _____ (present or absent).

Conclusion: _____

_____

ANALYSIS

RATE: 90 and 130/min. (normal and tachycardia). RHYTHM: irregular and supraventricular. P-R INTERVAL: 0.18 sec. (normal; constant). QRS DURATION: 0.09 sec. (normal). Q-T INTERVAL: 0.32 sec. (normal). P' WAVES: present.

Conclusion: This is a paroxysmal supraventricular tachycardia. It is sometimes called paroxysmal atrial tachycardia (PAT), paroxysmal A-V nodal tachycardia, reciprocating tachycardia, or A-V nodal reentry tachycardia. It begins abruptly with a PAC (the fourth P wave), after which it is thought that a reciprocating mechanism sustains the tachycardia.[47-51] This means that the PAC has caused one side of the A-V node to be out of phase with the other. That is, one side is depolarized while the other is still nonrefractory. The ventricles are captured normally; however, the impulse can now pass retrogradely (backward) up the A-V node through the nonrefractory pathway to depolarize the atria (atrial echo beat). By this time the other side of the A-V node is nonrefractory, and the stimulus passes antegradely (forward) down the node to recapture the ventricle (a reciprocal beat). This circuit continues around and around in the A-V node. It may be interrupted by a vagal maneuver or an appropriately timed stimulus. The atria may or may not be involved in the circuit. This is thought to be the most common mechanism of paroxysmal supraventricular tachycardia.

The two supraventricular tachycardias shown in the figure on p. 27 have rates in excess of 200/min. Surely this is a reciprocating mechanism, since the A-V node would usually block some of these impulses if it were not itself involved in the circuit.

Both a vagal maneuver and digitalis have been reported to successfully interrupt reciprocating rhythms by lengthening the refractory period of the A-V node.[52]

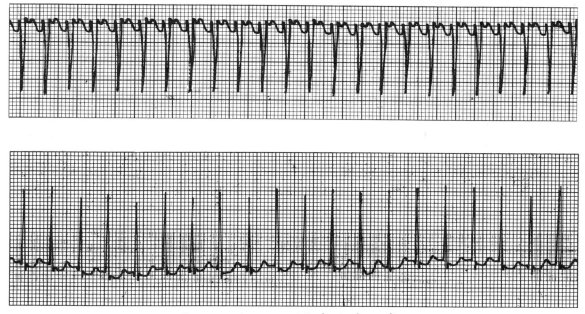

Paroxysmal supraventricular tachycardia.

EXERCISE 2-9

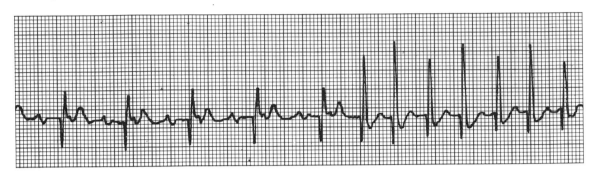

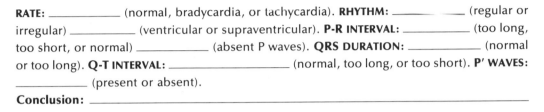

RATE: _____ (normal, bradycardia, or tachycardia). **RHYTHM:** _____ (regular or irregular) _____ (ventricular or supraventricular). **P-R INTERVAL:** _____ (too long, too short, or normal) _____ (absent P waves). **QRS DURATION:** _____ (normal or too long). **Q-T INTERVAL:** _____ (normal, too long, or too short). **P′ WAVES:** _____ (present or absent).

Conclusion: _____

_____

ANALYSIS

RATE: 86-172/min. (normal and tachycardia). **RHYTHM:** irregular and supraventricular. **P-R INTERVAL:** absent P waves. **QRS DURATION:** 0.08 sec. (normal). **Q-T INTERVAL:** 0.32 sec. (normal). **P′ WAVES:** present.

Conclusion: This is atrial tachycardia with 2:1 conduction in the first half of the tracing and 1:1 conduction in the last half. In the beginning of the tracing the ectopic P waves can be seen at a rate of 172/min. The conducted P′ wave is very evident before each ventricular complex (P′-R interval: 0.26 sec.). The nonconducted P′ follows the ventricular complex and distorts the T wave. It is helpful to remember that if P′ waves are in T waves, they will distort the T waves, *but usually the distortion will be different each time.* In other words, the P′ wave does not belong to the T wave but just happens to occur at the same time. Therefore, T waves that have P waves in them all usually look slightly different from each other.

When atrial tachycardia is accompanied by A-V block, the mechanism is probably not that of nodal reentry, because the blocked beat would interrupt the reentry circuit. Repeated firing of a single focus (enhanced automaticity) is more likely to be the mechanism in such a case.

EXERCISE 2-10

II

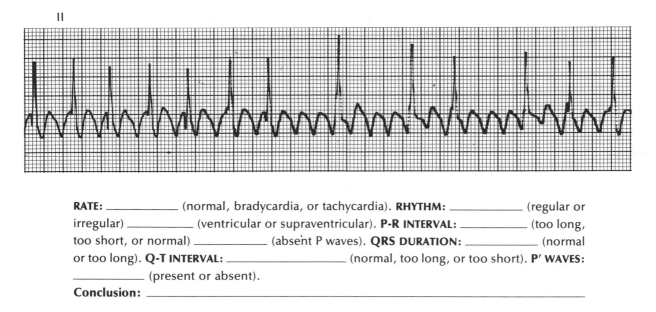

RATE: _____ (normal, bradycardia, or tachycardia). **RHYTHM:** _____ (regular or irregular) _____ (ventricular or supraventricular). **P-R INTERVAL:** _____ (too long, too short, or normal) _____ (absent P waves). **QRS DURATION:** _____ (normal or too long). **Q-T INTERVAL:** _____ (normal, too long, or too short). **P′ WAVES:** _____ (present or absent).

Conclusion: _____

_____

ANALYSIS

RATE: 80-150/min. (tachycardia). RHYTHM: irregular and supraventricular. **P-R INTERVAL:** absent P waves. **QRS DURATION:** 0.08 sec. (normal). **Q-T INTERVAL:** impossible to determine. **P′ WAVES:** present.

Conclusion: The typical sawtooth pattern of atrial flutter is unmistakable in this tracing. The atrial rate is 300/min. with variable block. In the beginning of the tracing the conduction ratio is 2:1, giving way to 4:1 and going back to 2:1.

This arrhythmia is thought to be the result of a reentry mechanism within the atrial conductive system.[56] It begins with one appropriately timed PAC and is easily terminated by cardioversion.

Notice that the P′ waves are right on time, with no pause to wait for the ventricular response. Atrial flutter is usually very easily spotted in the inferior leads (II, III, and aV$_F$) because of its typical distinguishing morphology. In these leads the P′ waves are the negative component and the Ta wave (atrial repolarization wave) is the positive component of the sawtooth pattern. In V$_1$ small upright P′ waves are usually seen. The twelve-lead ECG on p. 30 illustrates the changing faces of atrial flutter in the different leads. Notice V$_3$ and compare it with aV$_F$. There is 2:1 A-V conduction, which is easily seen in the inferior lead (aV$_F$) but is completely camouflaged in V$_3$. Sometimes, even in lead II, a 2:1 conduction is missed because one of the flutter waves is hidden in the QRS and T waves.

I   II   III

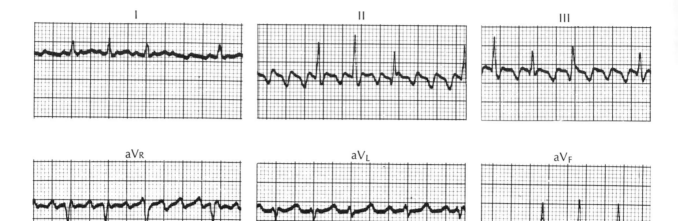

aV_R   aV_L   aV_F

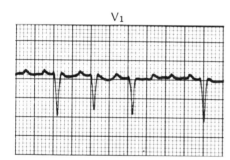
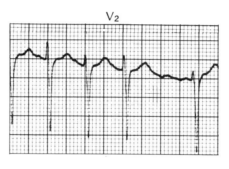
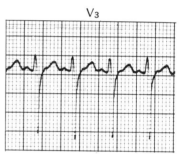

V_1   V_2   V_3

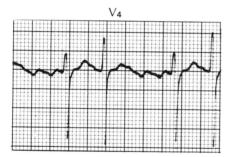
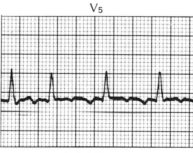
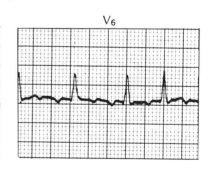

V_4   V_5   V_6

Atrial flutter.

EXERCISE 2-11

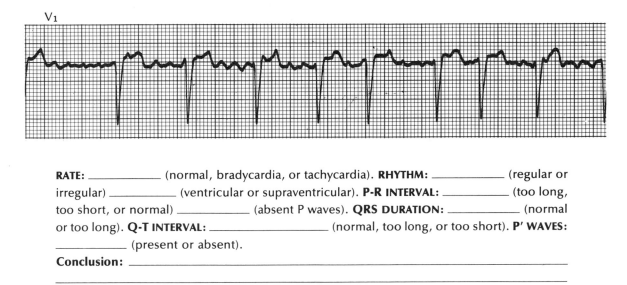

V₁

RATE: _____ (normal, bradycardia, or tachycardia). **RHYTHM:** _____ (regular or irregular) _____ (ventricular or supraventricular). **P-R INTERVAL:** _____ (too long, too short, or normal) _____ (absent P waves). **QRS DURATION:** _____ (normal or too long). **Q-T INTERVAL:** _____ (normal, too long, or too short). **P' WAVES:** _____ (present or absent).

Conclusion: _____

_____

ANALYSIS

RATE: 90-100/min. (normal). RHYTHM: irregular and supraventricular. P-R INTERVAL: absent P waves. QRS DURATION: 0.10 sec. (normal). Q-T INTERVAL: difficult to determine. P' WAVES: absent.

Conclusion: This is atrial fibrillation. Absent P waves and an irregular ventricular rhythm are the hallmarks of this arrhythmia. In this tracing there are some places that look like atrial flutter. The twelve leads shown in the preceding exercise should have convinced you that sometimes one lead is just not enough. This patient's ECG should also be checked in lead II. Remember that atrial flutter is absolutely regular through the tracing. By contrast, the tracing above has a very irregular fibrillatory line through it. This is caused by the erratic discharges within the atria. The irregular ventricular response is the result of concealed conduction. That is, some of the atrial stimuli only incompletely penetrate the A-V junction, leaving it refractory and resulting in an irregular ventricular rhythm.

EXERCISE 2-12

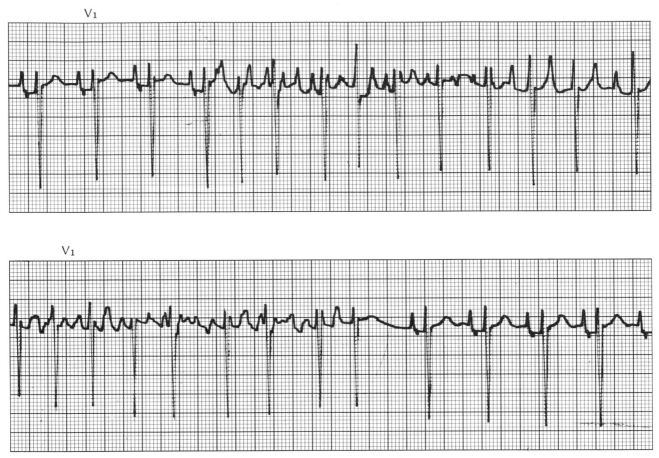

V₁

V₁

Same patient. Tracings not continuous.

RATE: _____ (normal, bradycardia, or tachycardia). **RHYTHM:** _____ (regular or irregular) _____ (ventricular or supraventricular). **P-R INTERVAL:** _____ (too long, too short, or normal) _____ (absent P waves). **QRS DURATION:** _____ (normal or too long). **Q-T INTERVAL:** _____ (normal, too long, or too short). **P' WAVES:** _____ (present or absent).

Conclusion: _____

_____

ANALYSIS

RATE: 100-140/min. (tachycardia). RHYTHM: irregular and supraventricular. P-R INTERVAL: 0.15 sec. (normal). QRS DURATION: 0.08 sec. (normal). Q-T INTERVAL: 0.32 sec. (normal). P' WAVES: present.

Conclusion: In this tracing atrial flutter and then fibrillation have resulted from a very short P-P' interval. The beginning of the tracing is a sinus rhythm of 100. The first P' wave is easily seen distorting the fourth T wave. Atrial flutter ensues, quickly deteriorating into atrial fibrillation. The second tracing shows the spontaneous conversion of atrial fibrillation into a normal sinus rhythm.

The hemodynamic consequences of a sudden onset of atrial fibrillation for the myocardial infarct patient can be very serious. Fibrillating atria do not pump blood. The atrial kick accounts for 20% of the cardiac output, a loss that an ischemic myocardium cannot afford.

EXERCISE 2-13

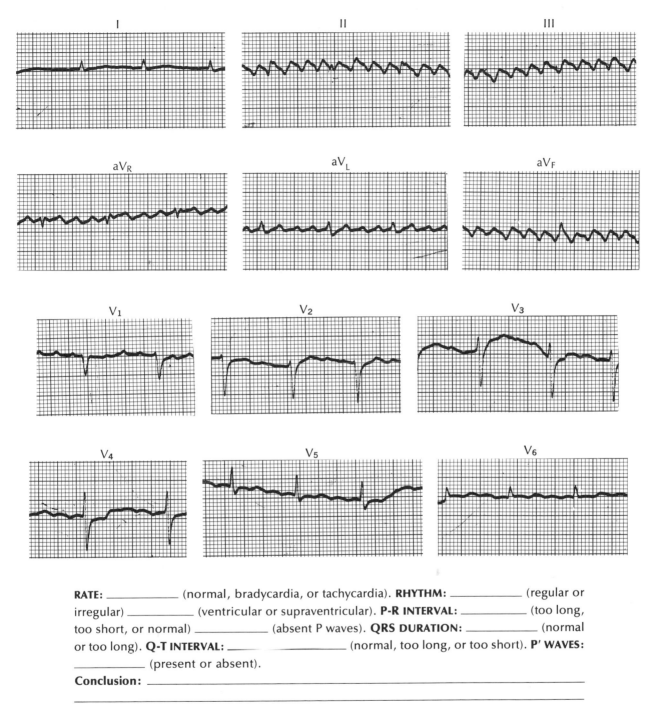

I	II	III
aV~R~	aV~L~	aV~F~
V₁	V₂	V₃
V₄	V₅	V₆

RATE: _____ (normal, bradycardia, or tachycardia). **RHYTHM:** _____ (regular or irregular) _____ (ventricular or supraventricular). **P-R INTERVAL:** _____ (too long, too short, or normal) _____ (absent P waves). **QRS DURATION:** _____ (normal or too long). **Q-T INTERVAL:** _____ _____ (normal, too long, or too short). **P' WAVES:** _____ (present or absent).

Conclusion: _____

_____

ANALYSIS

RATE: 80-84/min. (normal). RHYTHM: irregular and supraventricular. P-R INTERVAL: absent P waves. QRS DURATION: 0.08 sec. (normal). Q-T INTERVAL: impossible to determine. P' WAVES: present.

Conclusion: This is atrial flutter as seen in a twelve-lead ECG. Notice that in the inferior leads (II, III, and aV_F) the ventricular complex is barely detectable. This gives you an opportunity to notice the absolutely regular, uninterrupted cadence of the flutter waves. Notice that the P' waves are not seen at all in leads I, V_2, and V_3 in this particular patient, and yet atrial flutter is still present. In V_1 the P' waves are seen as little sharp peaks, much as a child would draw an ocean. In this lead the P' waves are not seen at all when the ventricular complex occurs. However, if you walk out the atrial rhythm, you will notice what looks like a little r' in the second ventricular complex. It is a P' wave.

This exercise has been included to convince you that when P waves are not seen in a tracing, one lead simply is not enough. The P vector may be isoelectric in the particular lead you are looking at. If such is the case, a flat line will be inscribed.

EXERCISE 2-14

V₁

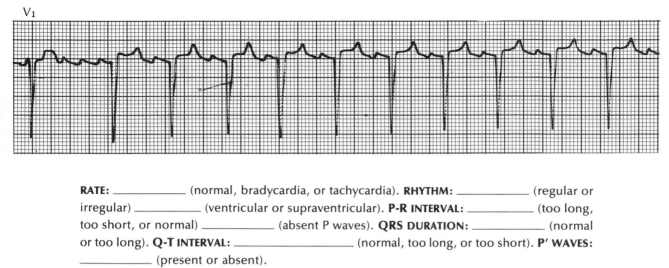

RATE: _____ (normal, bradycardia, or tachycardia). **RHYTHM:** _____ (regular or irregular) _____ (ventricular or supraventricular). **P-R INTERVAL:** _____ (too long, too short, or normal) _____ (absent P waves). **QRS DURATION:** _____ (normal or too long). **Q-T INTERVAL:** _____ (normal, too long, or too short). **P' WAVES:** _____ (present or absent).

Conclusion: _____

_____

ANALYSIS

RATE: 90-100/min. (normal). RHYTHM: irregular and supraventricular. P-R INTERVAL: absent P waves. QRS DURATION: 0.08 sec. (normal). Q-T INTERVAL: difficult to determine. P' WAVES: present.

Conclusion: This is an atrial flutter with an atrial rate of 300/min. and varying A-V conduction ratio. At the onset of the tracing the conduction ratio is 4:1. After that it is 3:1. Sometimes in atrial flutter when the conduction ratio is 2:1 or 3:1, the QRS-T will hide the flutter waves.

It is usually necessary to walk out the P' waves in order to determine the conduction ratio. Three P' waves in a row are easily seen at the beginning of the tracing. Place a piece of paper under these and mark them off. Then move the paper and mark the same ones again until you have about six or seven evenly spaced marks on your paper. Now place these marks across the ventricular complexes with the first mark on the P' wave preceding the QRS. You will see that there are three P' waves for every QRS. It is easy to see from this tracing that if only the last part of the tracing were available to you, you probably would not have diagnosed atrial flutter.

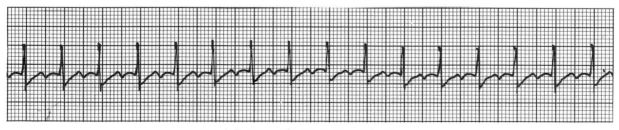
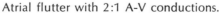

Atrial flutter with 2:1 A-V conductions.

In the figure above the conduction ratio is 2:1. It is a good rule to always suspect atrial flutter when the heart rate is around 150, as it is here.

EXERCISE 2-15

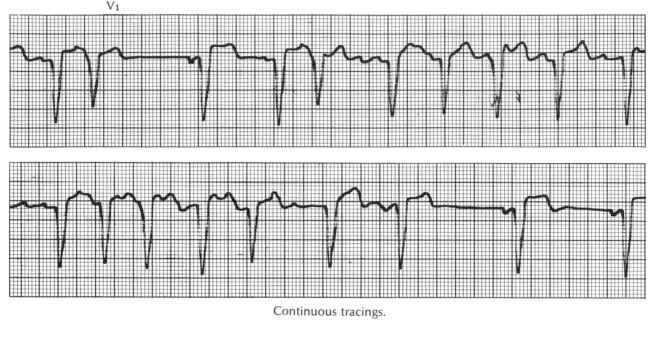

Continuous tracings.

RATE: _____ (normal, bradycardia, or tachycardia). **RHYTHM:** _____ (regular or irregular) _____ (ventricular or supraventricular). **P-R INTERVAL:** _____ (too long, too short, or normal) _____ (absent P waves). **QRS DURATION:** _____ (normal or too long). **Q-T INTERVAL:** _____ (normal, too long, or too short). **P' WAVES:** _____ (present or absent).

Conclusion: _____

_____

ANALYSIS

RATE: 55-110/min. (tachycardia). RHYTHM: irregular and supraventricular. P-R INTERVAL: 0.12 sec. (normal). QRS DURATION: 0.12 sec. (too long). Q-T INTERVAL: 0.40 sec. (normal). P' WAVES: present.

Conclusion: This patient has frequent PACs, which eventually produce a paroxysm of atrial fibrillation. The tracing begins with two PACs, followed by a normal sinus beat and two more PACs. This time the second P' in the group produces atrial fibrillation. Here again, as in exercise 2-12, a short P-P' interval results in electrical disunity in the atria and atrial fibrillation. In the second strip the arrhythmia is seen to spontaneously convert into a normal sinus rhythm.

The patient's main electrocardiographic problem is that of sinus bradycardia and PACs. In this case the atrial fibrillation is simply a result of the PAC. As mentioned in exercise 2-12, a paroxysm of atrial fibrillation causes a sudden fall in cardiac output and coronary perfusion. It is, therefore, important to protect this patient from further bouts of atrial fibrillation. It may only be necessary to ensure adequate oxygenation. The electrolyte panel should be checked, and a third heart sound should be listened for, since PACs are also an early sign of congestive heart failure.

EXERCISE 2-16

V₁

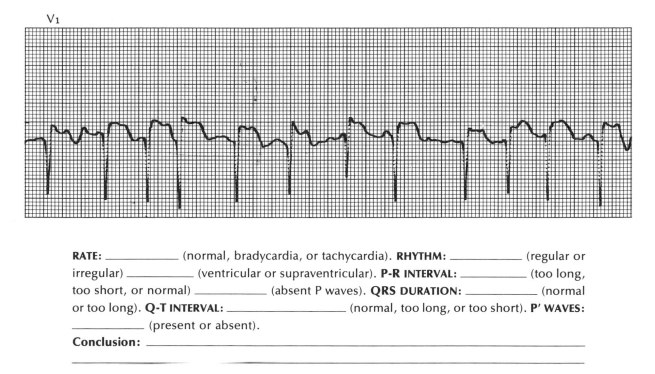

RATE: _____ (normal, bradycardia, or tachycardia). **RHYTHM:** _____ (regular or irregular) _____ (ventricular or supraventricular). **P-R INTERVAL:** _____ (too long, too short, or normal) _____ (absent P waves). **QRS DURATION:** _____ (normal or too long). **Q-T INTERVAL:** _____ (normal, too long, or too short). **P' WAVES:** _____ (present or absent).

Conclusion: _____

ANALYSIS

RATE: 110-130/min. (tachycardia). RHYTHM: irregular and supraventricular. P-R INTERVAL: absent P waves. QRS DURATION: 0.06 sec. (normal). Q-T INTERVAL: impossible to determine. P' WAVES: absent.

Conclusion: This is atrial fibrillation. The grossly irregular ventricular rhythm is what you would expect in this arrhythmia. The rate indicates that it is uncontrolled (not adequately treated).

The drug of choice in the treatment of atrial fibrillation is digitalis. It is used to slow the ventricular rate. Digitalis lengthens the refractory period at the A-V node, limiting the number of impulses that can penetrate. Since there is no P-R interval to gauge the effect of the digitalis on A-V conduction, you must pay special attention to any regularization of the ventricular rhythm. Remember that in atrial fibrillation the ventricular response *should* be absolutely irregular. If heart block is present, a junctional pacemaker will pace the ventricles. This pacemaker will be protected from the chaotic activity in the atria by the block, which may be either complete or intermittent. The ventricular rhythm will then be absolutely regular, or intermittent regularity will be seen in the case of incomplete block. Digitalis, if given in excess, will cause heart block and may also result in junctional tachycardia.

The figure on p. 38 is an example of atrial fibrillation and complete heart block. The fibrillatory line is clearly seen through the tracing. However, the ventricular rhythm is absolutely regular at approximately 47/min. This indicates complete heart block. This patient has not received digitalis; therefore, it is a pathological block and is not drug induced.

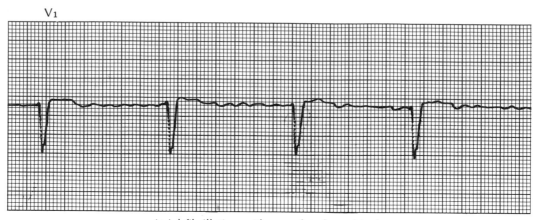

V_1

Atrial fibrillation with complete heart block.

EXERCISE 2-17

V₁

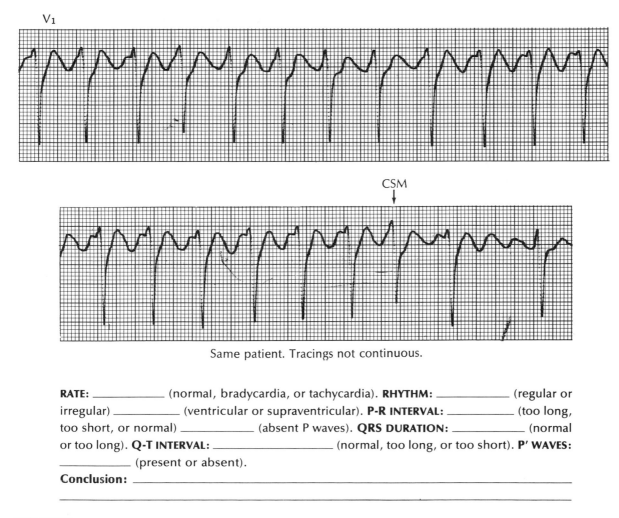

CSM

Same patient. Tracings not continuous.

RATE: _____ (normal, bradycardia, or tachycardia). **RHYTHM:** _____ (regular or irregular) _____ (ventricular or supraventricular). **P-R INTERVAL:** _____ (too long, too short, or normal) _____ (absent P waves). **QRS DURATION:** _____ (normal or too long). **Q-T INTERVAL:** _____ (normal, too long, or too short). **P′ WAVES:** _____ (present or absent).

Conclusion: _____

_____

ANALYSIS

RATE: 110-112/min. (tachycardia). RHYTHM: irregular and supraventricular. P-R INTERVAL: absent P waves. QRS DURATION: 0.12 sec. (too long). Q-T INTERVAL: difficult to determine. P′ WAVES: present.

Conclusion: In the first tracing there are no distinct P waves. The changing shape in front of the r waves should cause you to suspect the hidden flutter wave (atrial flutter with 2:1 block). This diagnosis is confirmed in the second tracing from the same patient where a 4:1 conduction ratio is seen in response to carotid sinus massage (CSM). Clearly seen at the end of the tracing is the undulating pattern of atrial flutter. However, the atrial rate is only 220-224/min. Some authorities would call this an atrial tachycardia and say that it would be an atrial flutter only if the atrial rate exceeded 250/min. Others would say that no matter what the rate, a sawtooth pattern is atrial flutter. No matter what it is called, the main consideration is that a rapid ventricular rate has resulted from an ectopic atrial tachycardia.

EXERCISE 2-18

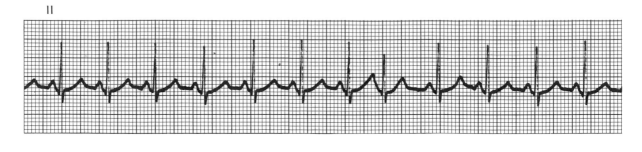

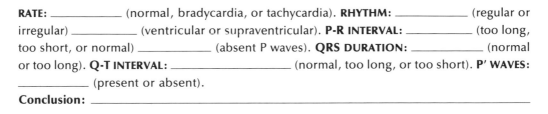

RATE: _____ (normal, bradycardia, or tachycardia). **RHYTHM:** _____ (regular or irregular) _____ (ventricular or supraventricular). **P-R INTERVAL:** _____ (too long, too short, or normal) _____ (absent P waves). **QRS DURATION:** _____ (normal or too long). **Q-T INTERVAL:** _____ (normal, too long, or too short). **P' WAVES:** _____ (present or absent).

Conclusion: _____

_____

ANALYSIS

RATE: 118/min. (tachycardia). **RHYTHM:** irregular and supraventricular. **P-R INTERVAL:** 0.10 sec. (normal). **QRS DURATION:** 0.08 sec. (normal). **Q-T INTERVAL:** 0.28 sec. (normal). **P' WAVES:** present.

Conclusion: This is a sinus tachycardia. The single irregularity in the tracing is caused by a PAC. This P' wave is hidden in a T wave in approximately the middle of the strip. It causes the T wave to be tall and peaked.

Sinus tachycardia in a resting patient and PACs are both signs of congestive heart failure. They are not conclusive signs but should make you aware of a possible problem.

EXERCISE 2-19

V₁

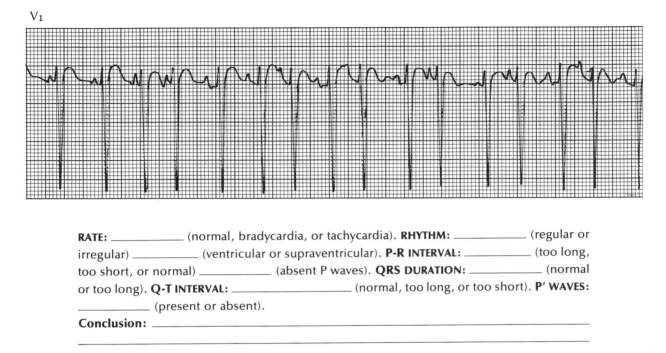

RATE: _____ (normal, bradycardia, or tachycardia). **RHYTHM:** _____ (regular or irregular) _____ (ventricular or supraventricular). **P-R INTERVAL:** _____ (too long, too short, or normal) _____ (absent P waves). **QRS DURATION:** _____ (normal or too long). **Q-T INTERVAL:** _____ (normal, too long, or too short). **P′ WAVES:** _____ (present or absent).

Conclusion: _____

_____

ANALYSIS

RATE: 140-160/min. (tachycardia). RHYTHM: irregular and supraventricular. P-R INTER-VAL: difficult to determine P waves (many P′ waves are evident). QRS DURATION: 0.08 sec. (normal). Q-T INTERVAL: 0.25 sec. (normal). P′ WAVES: present.

Conclusion: This tracing represents chaotic atrial tachycardia or multifocal PACs. Because there are so many P′ waves occurring, it is difficult to tell if there are any sinus P waves at all. This arrhythmia is said to often accompany pulmonary disease and electrolyte imbalance.

EXERCISE 2-20

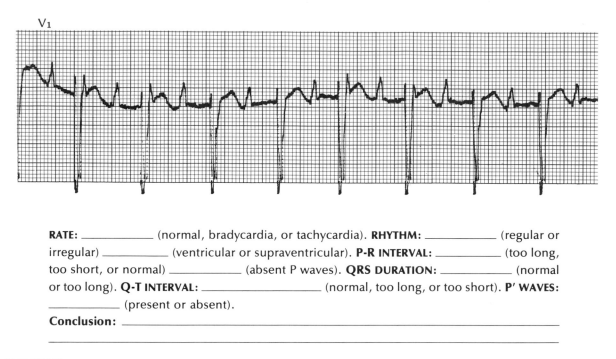

V₁

RATE: _____ (normal, bradycardia, or tachycardia). **RHYTHM:** _____ (regular or irregular) _____ (ventricular or supraventricular). **P-R INTERVAL:** _____ (too long, too short, or normal) _____ (absent P waves). **QRS DURATION:** _____ (normal or too long). **Q-T INTERVAL:** _____ (normal, too long, or too short). **P' WAVES:** _____ (present or absent).

Conclusion: _____

_____

ANALYSIS

RATE: 84/min. (normal). RHYTHM: regular and supraventricular. P-R INTERVAL: absent P waves. QRS DURATION: 0.10 sec. (normal). Q-T INTERVAL: 0.32 sec. (normal). P' WAVES: present.

Conclusion: This is an atrial tachycardia with 2:1 A-V conduction. A slight somatic tremor runs through the tracing, but it is not enough to preclude a diagnosis. Notice that some of the ventricular complexes have an R' wave, whereas others do not. That "R'" wave is really a P' partially hidden by the ventricular complex. If you happened to use the QRS with this distortion to measure your QRS duration, you will have an incorrect and abnormally long measurement.

Whenever P waves are midway between two R waves, it is wise to always suspect a hidden P (Killip's rule), which is the case here. If the hidden P had not been noticed, a diagnosis of first-degree heart block would have been made, when the patient really has an atrial tachycardia of 168/min. with 2:1 A-V conduction. This arrhythmia suggests a mechanism of enhanced automaticity in the atrium or reentry above the A-V node. A-V block is thought to rule out an A-V nodal reentry mechanism. The occurrence of block during reciprocal A-V nodal tachycardia is thought to be rare.[53]

EXERCISE 2-21

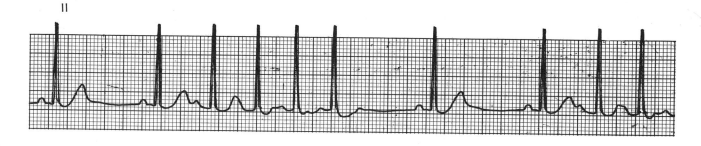

II

RATE: _____ (normal, bradycardia, or tachycardia). **RHYTHM:** _____ (regular or irregular) _____ (ventricular or supraventricular). **P-R INTERVAL:** _____ (too long, too short, or normal) _____ (absent P waves). **QRS DURATION:** _____ (normal or too long). **Q-T INTERVAL:** _____ (normal, too long, or too short). **P' WAVES:** _____ (present or absent).

Conclusion: _____

_____

ANALYSIS

RATE: 56-175/min. (bradycardia and tachycardia). RHYTHM: irregular and supraventricular. P-R INTERVAL: 0.16 sec. (normal). QRS DURATION: 0.06 sec. (normal). Q-T INTERVAL: 0.40 sec. with the bradycardia (normal). P' WAVES: present.

Conclusion: This is PAT. The underlying rhythm is a sinus bradycardia of 56/min. The supraventricular tachycardia begins with a PAC after the second R wave. It terminates and then begins again after two more sinus beats. This arrhythmia is thought to be an A-V nodal reentry mechanism. It usually requires no treatment, is self-limiting, and can be terminated by a vagal maneuver.

EXERCISE 2-22

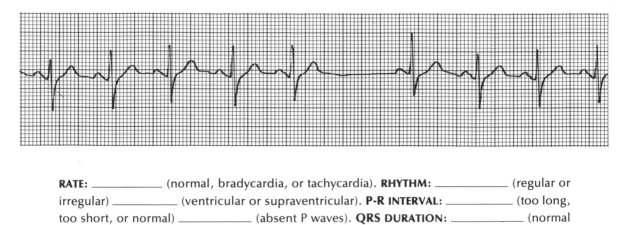

RATE: _____ (normal, bradycardia, or tachycardia). **RHYTHM:** _____ (regular or irregular) _____ (ventricular or supraventricular). **P-R INTERVAL:** _____ (too long, too short, or normal) _____ (absent P waves). **QRS DURATION:** _____ (normal or too long). **Q-T INTERVAL:** _____ (normal, too long, or too short). **P' WAVES:** _____ (present or absent).

Conclusion: _____

_____

ANALYSIS

RATE: 92/min. (underlying rate normal). RHYTHM: irregular and supraventricular. **P-R INTERVAL:** 0.14 sec. (normal). **QRS DURATION:** 0.08 sec. (normal). **Q-T INTERVAL:** 0.32 sec. (normal). **P' WAVES:** present.

Conclusion: This is probably a nonconducted PAC. The T wave preceding the pause is only slightly distorted. However, there is a slowing of the sinus rhythm after the pause. A PAC would cause such a suppression. Also, sinus exit block is far less frequent. Statistics alone would favor the nonconducted PAC.

In this tracing you have another opportunity to notice how the length of the refractory period changes with heart rate. Notice the difference between the Q-T interval preceding the pause and that of the one following it. As the length of the cycle increases, the refractory period also increases.

EXERCISE 2-23

V₁

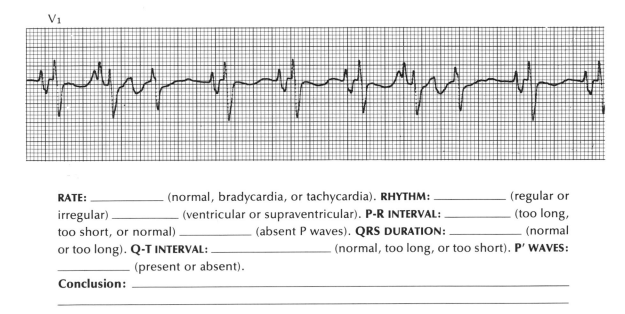

RATE: _____ (normal, bradycardia, or tachycardia). **RHYTHM:** _____ (regular or irregular) _____ (ventricular or supraventricular). **P-R INTERVAL:** _____ (too long, too short, or normal) _____ (absent P waves). **QRS DURATION:** _____ (normal or too long). **Q-T INTERVAL:** _____ (normal, too long, or too short). **P' WAVES:** _____ (present or absent).

Conclusion: _____

_____

ANALYSIS

RATE: 84/min. (underlying rate normal). RHYTHM: irregular and supraventricular. P-R INTERVAL: 0.16 sec. (normal). QRS DURATION: 0.10 sec. (normal). Q-T INTERVAL: 0.38 sec. (too long). P' WAVES: present.

Conclusion: There are P' waves in this tracing. Two are very apparent. They precede the second and the seventh beats and are normally conducted. Notice the T wave following the first PAC of the group. It is distorted with another P' wave (an atrial echo beat) and the potential beginning of a reciprocating mechanism. A ventricular complex follows then another atrial echo beat. This is where the mechanism stops, at least for the moment. This patient later continued with the reciprocating mechanism and aberrant ventricular conduction.

EXERCISE 2-24

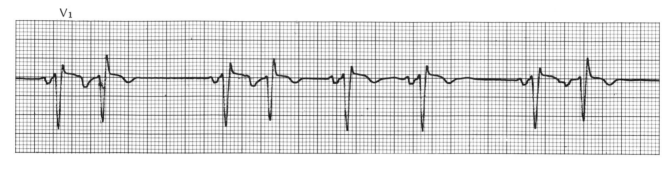

V$_1$

RATE: _____ (normal, bradycardia, or tachycardia). **RHYTHM:** _____ (regular or irregular) _____ (ventricular or supraventricular). **P-R INTERVAL:** _____ (too long, too short, or normal) _____ (absent P waves). **QRS DURATION:** _____ (normal or too long). **Q-T INTERVAL:** _____ (normal, too long, or too short). **P' WAVES:** _____ (present or absent).

Conclusion: _____

_____

ANALYSIS

RATE: approximately 80/min. (normal). **RHYTHM:** irregular and supraventricular. **P-R INTERVAL:** 0.12 sec. (normal). **QRS DURATION:** 0.12 sec. (too long). **Q-T INTERVAL:** 0.40 sec. (too long). **P' WAVES:** present.

Conclusion: There are three PACs in this tracing. They occur coupled to the first, second, and last sinus beats. The underlying rhythm is sinus arrhythmia. When you examine such an irregular tracing, try to find two sinus beats in a row and more, if possible. When you evaluate any arrhythmia, determine if the sinus node has a normal rate and rhythm. In this tracing there are three sinus P waves, which are consecutive, beginning in the middle of the tracing (fifth complex). In this group you will find the only two T waves that you can be sure do not have P' waves in them. If you compare their shape with the other T waves, you will easily find the PACs. Bigeminal PACs begin after a pause in the sinus rhythm.

The broad triphasic pattern in V$_1$ is indicative of right bundle branch block. This is discussed along with the exercises in Chapter 6.

EXERCISE 2-25

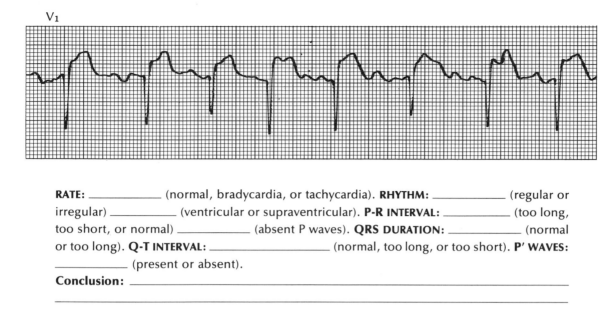

V₁

RATE: _____ (normal, bradycardia, or tachycardia). **RHYTHM:** _____ (regular or irregular) _____ (ventricular or supraventricular). **P-R INTERVAL:** _____ (too long, too short, or normal) _____ (absent P waves). **QRS DURATION:** _____ (normal or too long). **Q-T INTERVAL:** _____ (normal, too long, or too short). **P′ WAVES:** _____ (present or absent).

Conclusion: _____

_____

ANALYSIS

RATE: 75-85/min. (normal). **RHYTHM:** irregular and supraventricular. **P-R INTERVAL:** absent P waves. **QRS DURATION:** 0.07 sec. (normal). **Q-T INTERVAL:** difficult to determine. **P′ WAVES:** absent.

Conclusion: This is atrial fibrillation. However, there is too much regularization. That is, too many cycle lengths are exactly the same. This is one of the first signs in atrial fibrillation of digitalis toxicity.

EXERCISE 2-26

V₁

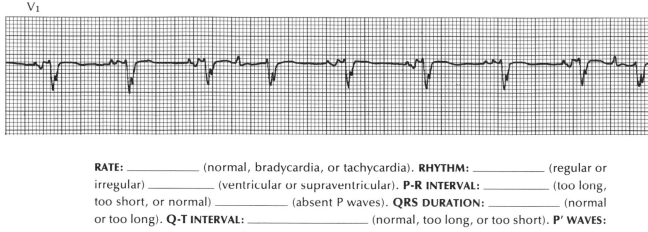

RATE: _____ (normal, bradycardia, or tachycardia). **RHYTHM:** _____ (regular or irregular) _____ (ventricular or supraventricular). **P-R INTERVAL:** _____ (too long, too short, or normal) _____ (absent P waves). **QRS DURATION:** _____ (normal or too long). **Q-T INTERVAL:** _____ (normal, too long, or too short). **P′ WAVES:** _____ (present or absent).

Conclusion: _____

_____

ANALYSIS

RATE: 75-80/min. (normal). **RHYTHM:** irregular and supraventricular. **P-R INTERVAL:** 0.16 sec. (normal). **QRS DURATION:** 0.10 sec. (normal). **Q-T INTERVAL:** 0.32 sec. (too short). **P′ WAVES:** present.

Conclusion: There are two P′ waves in this tracing. They precede the fourth and last ventricular complexes and are easily seen because of their prematurity and different shape. The sinus P waves have a double hump and, although they are right on time, vary in morphology. This may be due to atrial fusion. That is, a PAC may have occurred at the same time as the sinus node discharge and produced a collision of electrical forces, or it may simply be the result of patient movement or respiration.

Please note the length of the P′-R intervals. They are both noticeably longer than the P-R intervals. This is because the P′ wave occurred so close to the preceding T wave that the A-V junction was still refractory, causing a delay in conduction.

A P′-R interval may also be shorter than the P-R interval, as would occur when the atrial ectopic focus is low in the right atria close to the A-V node.

EXERCISE 2-27

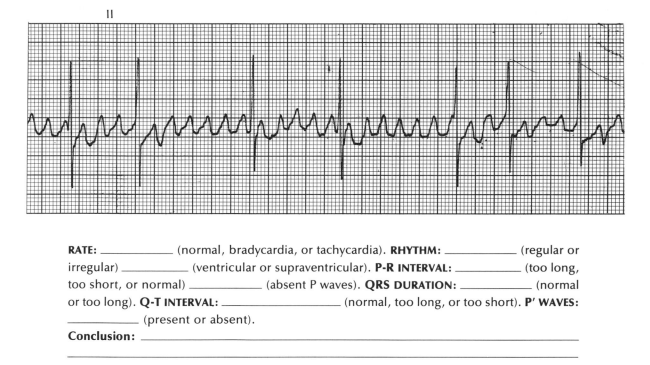

II

RATE: _____ (normal, bradycardia, or tachycardia). **RHYTHM:** _____ (regular or irregular) _____ (ventricular or supraventricular). **P-R INTERVAL:** _____ (too long, too short, or normal) _____ (absent P waves). **QRS DURATION:** _____ (normal or too long). **Q-T INTERVAL:** _____ (normal, too long, or too short). **P' WAVES:** _____ (present or absent).

Conclusion: _____

_____

ANALYSIS

RATE: 65-70/min. (normal). **RHYTHM:** irregular and supraventricular. **P-R INTERVAL:** absent P waves. **QRS DURATION:** 0.07 sec. (normal). **Q-T INTERVAL:** impossible to determine. **P' WAVES:** present.

Conclusion: This is atrial flutter with variable A-V conduction. The atrial rate here is 300/min., with anywhere from two to seven P waves for every QRS complex. With a 7:1 conduction ratio, some degree of A-V heart block would be suspected.

EXERCISE 2-28

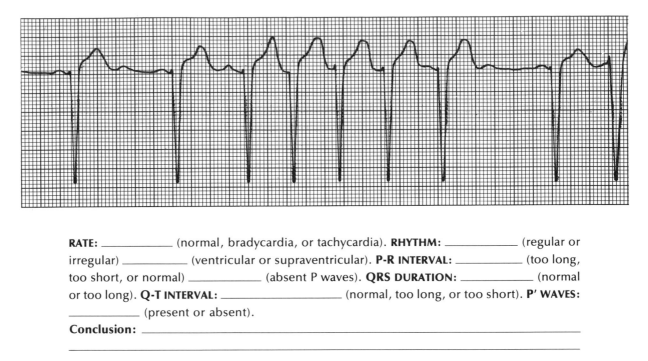

RATE: _____ (normal, bradycardia, or tachycardia). **RHYTHM:** _____ (regular or irregular) _____ (ventricular or supraventricular). **P-R INTERVAL:** _____ (too long, too short, or normal) _____ (absent P waves). **QRS DURATION:** _____ (normal or too long). **Q-T INTERVAL:** _____ (normal, too long, or too short). **P' WAVES:** _____ (present or absent).

Conclusion: _____

_____

ANALYSIS

RATE: 55-125/min. (tachycardia). **P-R INTERVAL:** 0.14 sec. (normal). **QRS DURATION:** 0.12 sec. (too long). **Q-T INTERVAL:** 0.42 sec. with the bradycardia (normal). **P' WAVES:** present.

Conclusion: Here again is an example of PAT. The tracing begins with two sinus P waves. A prominent U wave is present. This is usually a sign of hypokalemia, which may have caused the PACs. A P' wave follows the second complex, and a paroxysm of supraventricular tachycardia ensues. It terminates spontaneously, only to begin again after one normal sinus beat.

EXERCISE 2-29

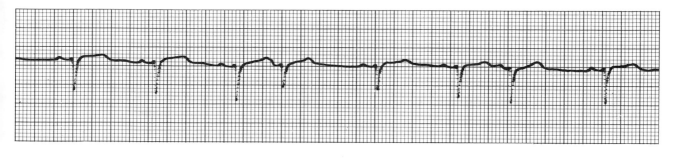

RATE: _____ (normal, bradycardia, or tachycardia). **RHYTHM:** _____ (regular or irregular) _____ (ventricular or supraventricular). **P-R INTERVAL:** _____ (too long, too short, or normal) _____ (absent P waves). **QRS DURATION:** _____ (normal or too long). **Q-T INTERVAL:** _____ (normal, too long, or too short). **P′ WAVES:** _____ (present or absent).

Conclusion: _____
_____

ANALYSIS

RATE: 70-80/min. (normal). **RHYTHM:** irregular and supraventricular. **P-R INTERVAL:** 0.14 sec. (normal). **QRS DURATION:** 0.08 sec. (normal). **Q-T INTERVAL:** 0.38 sec. (normal). **P′ WAVES:** present.

Conclusion: The irregularity in the above rhythm is caused by PACs occurring after the third and sixth beats. The first P′ wave is buried in a T wave. The second P′ wave falls after a T wave, looking almost like a U wave.

EXERCISE 2-30

V₁

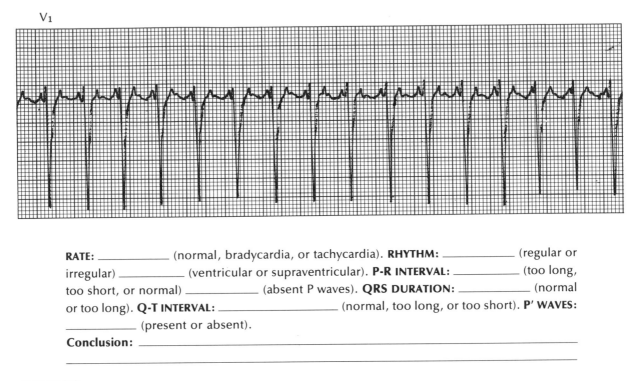

RATE: _____ (normal, bradycardia, or tachycardia). **RHYTHM:** _____ (regular or irregular) _____ (ventricular or supraventricular). **P-R INTERVAL:** _____ (too long, too short, or normal) _____ (absent P waves). **QRS DURATION:** _____ (normal or too long). **Q-T INTERVAL:** _____ (normal, too long, or too short). **P' WAVES:** _____ (present or absent).

Conclusion: _____

_____

ANALYSIS

RATE: 150/min. (tachycardia). **RHYTHM:** regular and supraventricular. **P-R INTERVAL:** absent P waves. **QRS DURATION:** 0.09 sec. (normal). **Q-T INTERVAL:** 0.26 sec. (normal). **P' WAVES:** present.

Conclusion: There are two P' waves for every QRS complex. The atrial rate is 300/min. In lead II you would see the sawtooth pattern of atrial flutter, which often goes undetected when the conduction ratio is 2:1, as it is here. In lead V₁ above, the P' waves are easily seen just before the ventricular complex and in the S-T segment.

Cardioversion is usually very effective in terminating this arrhythmia.

CHAPTER 3
JUNCTIONAL ECTOPICS

Chapters 2 and 3 are closely linked because atrial and junctional ectopic rhythms often have the same clinical implications, treatment, and ECG morphology. In fact, given the credence of the A-V nodal reentry mechanism (Chapter 2), paroxysmal junctional tachycardia and PAT are the same.

Junctional ectopic beats are recognized because the ventricular complex is of the same morphology as the sinus conducted beats. The P′ wave resulting from the discharge of pacemaker cells within the A-V junction may or may not be seen. If it is seen, it will be either immediately before the QRS, with a P′-R interval of less than 0.11 sec., or it will follow the QRS. In both cases it is usually negative in the inferior leads (II, III, and aV$_F$).[63] In addition, there may be retrograde block from the junctional focus and therefore no P′ wave.

In the case of junctional tachycardia the mechanism becomes an important part of the diagnostic process. Paroxysmal junctional tachycardia is generally thought to be the result of a reentry circuit within the A-V node. It usually ends spontaneously and requires no treatment. However, *non*paroxysmal junctional tachycardia is the result of enhanced automaticity, which may have been caused by digitalis excess and requires withdrawal of the drug.

This chapter deals with isolated premature junctional beats, reciprocating A-V junctional tachycardia (PAT), nonparoxysmal junctional tachycardia, and junctional escape beats and rhythms. This chapter also includes examples of A-V dissociation, which is the result of either junctional tachycardia or a junctional escape mechanism responding to another arrhythmia, usually sinus bradycardia.

EXERCISE 3-1

V₁

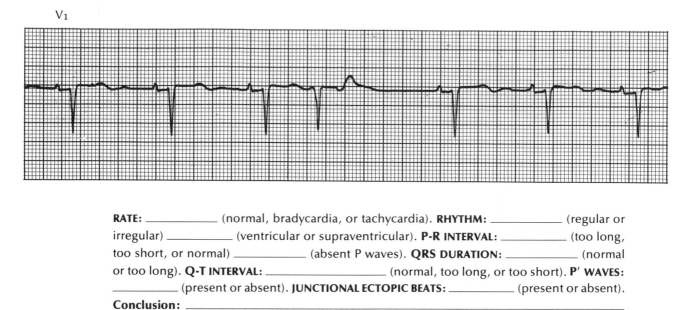

RATE: _____ (normal, bradycardia, or tachycardia). **RHYTHM:** _____ (regular or irregular) _____ (ventricular or supraventricular). **P-R INTERVAL:** _____ (too long, too short, or normal) _____ (absent P waves). **QRS DURATION:** _____ (normal or too long). **Q-T INTERVAL:** _____ (normal, too long, or too short). **P′ WAVES:** _____ (present or absent). **JUNCTIONAL ECTOPIC BEATS:** _____ (present or absent).

Conclusion: _____

_____

ANALYSIS

RATE: 60-65/min. (normal). RHYTHM: irregular and supraventricular. P-R INTERVAL: 0.15 sec. (normal). QRS DURATION: 0.08 sec. (normal). Q-T INTERVAL: 0.40 sec. (normal). P′ WAVES: present. JUNCTIONAL ECTOPIC BEATS: present.

Conclusion: This tracing contains a premature junctional contraction (PJC). The fourth complex is clearly the same morphology as the preceding sinus conducted beats. It is therefore supraventricular in origin. Close examination of the T wave preceding the premature beat reveals no distortion. It can therefore be assumed that this ectopic focus is in the A-V junction. The distortion in the T wave of the premature beat is caused by retrograde activation of the atria from the junctional ectopic focus.

When measuring the P-R interval in this tracing, you may not have noticed the tiny r wave preceding the S. If you did not, then your P-R interval would have been slightly too long and your QRS duration would have been too short for the same reason.

Note the U wave in this tracing. It is the extra hump following the T wave and is normally the same polarity as the T wave. A prominent U wave is a sensitive indicator of hypokalemia and is best seen in V₃. Usually the U wave is closer to the T wave and in the case of hypokalemia becomes more prominent, causing the Q-T interval to appear prolonged (flattened and widened). Untreated hypokalemia will give way to T wave inversion and sagging S-T segment.

EXERCISE 3-2

V₁

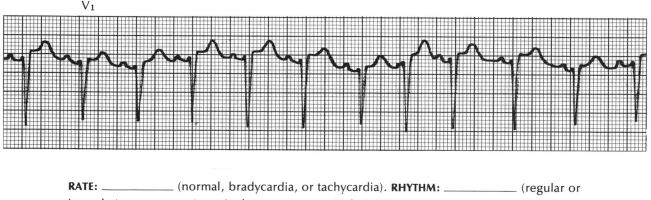

RATE: _____ (normal, bradycardia, or tachycardia). **RHYTHM:** _____ (regular or irregular) _____ (ventricular or supraventricular). **P-R INTERVAL:** _____ (too long, too short, or normal) _____ (absent P waves). **QRS DURATION:** _____ (normal or too long). **Q-T INTERVAL:** _____ (normal, too long, or too short). **P' WAVES:** _____ (present or absent). **JUNCTIONAL ECTOPIC BEATS:** _____ (present or absent).

Conclusion: _____

_____

ANALYSIS

RATE: 92-100/min. (normal). RHYTHM: irregular and supraventricular. P-R INTERVAL: 0.14 sec. (normal). QRS DURATION: 0.10 sec. (normal). Q-T INTERVAL: 0.32 sec. (normal). P' WAVES: present. JUNCTIONAL ECTOPIC BEATS: present.

Conclusion: The single irregularity in this tracing is due to a premature junctional ectopic beat. If you walk out the P waves, you will find that the eighth complex is premature.

It is a matter of interest and not clinically important whether or not a junctional ectopic focus has conducted retrogradely to the atria. In the past the location of the P' wave before, during, or after the ventricular complex was stressed. This is because it was thought that such information was an indicator of the precise site of the ectopic focus. It is now known that the location of the P' wave is also a function of conduction velocity and therefore does not determine location.

In the tracing above, the P' wave can be seen just before the eighth QRS complex (a sharp little peak distorting the r wave). The P'-R interval is 0.04 sec.

EXERCISE 3-3

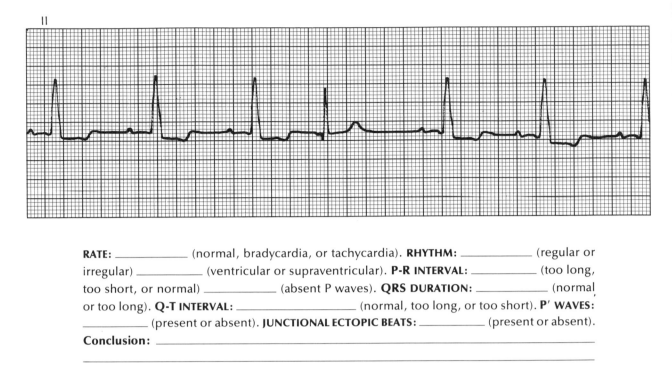

II

RATE: _____ (normal, bradycardia, or tachycardia). **RHYTHM:** _____ (regular or irregular) _____ (ventricular or supraventricular). **P-R INTERVAL:** _____ (too long, too short, or normal) _____ (absent P waves). **QRS DURATION:** _____ (normal or too long). **Q-T INTERVAL:** _____ (normal, too long, or too short). **P′ WAVES:** _____ (present or absent). **JUNCTIONAL ECTOPIC BEATS:** _____ (present or absent).

Conclusion: _____

_____

ANALYSIS

RATE: 56/min. (bradycardia). RHYTHM: irregular and supraventricular. P-R INTERVAL: 0.24 sec. (too long). QRS DURATION: 0.10 sec. (normal). Q-T INTERVAL: 0.42 sec. (normal). P′ WAVES: present (hidden). JUNCTIONAL ECTOPIC BEATS: present.

Conclusion: The PJC in this tracing appears to be narrower than the sinus-conducted beats. It sometimes happens that a junctional ectopic focus is a little offset within the A-V junction. Therefore, the wave front resulting from this stimulus will not be exactly the same as the more unifom one generated by the sinus-conducted impulse. This can cause the junctional beat, even a late one, to be a little aberrant.[61,62]

In this tracing there is retrograde conduction to the atria, evidenced by the P′ wave in front of the junctional ectopic beat (P′-R interval: 0.06 sec.). You will notice that there is a less than full compensatory pause. This in itself indicates premature firing of the sinus node from an ectopic focus.

Sinus bradycardia and first-degree heart block are also noted in this tracing. The latter diagnosis is made by measuring the P-R interval and finding it to be greater than 0.20 sec. This is discussed more fully in Chapter 5.

EXERCISE 3-4

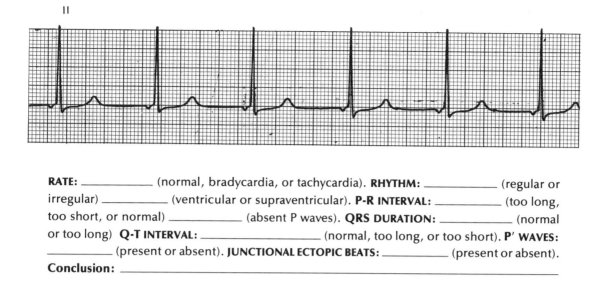

II

RATE: _____ (normal, bradycardia, or tachycardia). **RHYTHM:** _____ (regular or irregular) _____ (ventricular or supraventricular). **P-R INTERVAL:** _____ (too long, too short, or normal) _____ (absent P waves). **QRS DURATION:** _____ (normal or too long) **Q-T INTERVAL:** _____ (normal, too long, or too short). **P′ WAVES:** _____ (present or absent). **JUNCTIONAL ECTOPIC BEATS:** _____ (present or absent).
Conclusion: _____

ANALYSIS

RATE: 58/min. (bradycardia). **RHYTHM:** regular and supraventricular. **P-R INTERVAL:** absent P waves. **QRS DURATION:** 0.08 sec. (normal). **Q-T INTERVAL:** 0.48 sec. (too long). **P′ WAVES:** present. **JUNCTIONAL ECTOPIC BEATS:** present.

Conclusion: This is a junctional escape rhythm. In lead II a negative P′ wave and short P′-R interval (less than 0.12 sec.) are two indicators of an ectopic junctional pacemaker. The P′-R interval in this case is 0.08 sec., and the ventricular complexes are clearly supraventricular. The rate is compatible with the inherent rate of the A-V junctional pacemaker cells, qualifying this as a passive escape mechanism as opposed to an active mechanism. The pacemaker cells in the A-V junction will usually escape and pace the heart if the sinus node fails to do so.

The treatment of this arrhythmia will depend on the hemodynamic state of the patient. The junctional escape rhythm itself will not be treated. If the patient is hypotensive, it may be necessary to increase the rate of the sinus node with atropine. (Refer to the discussion on p. 9.)

EXERCISE   3-5

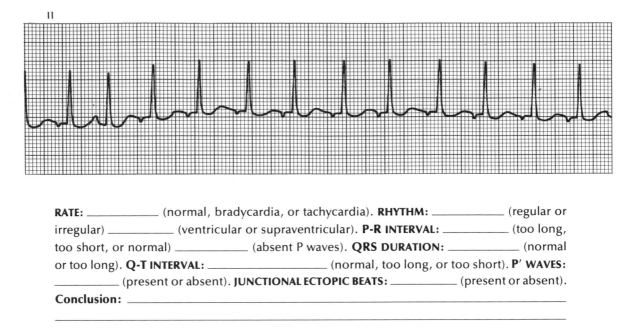

II

RATE: _____ (normal, bradycardia, or tachycardia). **RHYTHM:** _____ (regular or irregular) _____ (ventricular or supraventricular). **P-R INTERVAL:** _____ (too long, too short, or normal) _____ (absent P waves). **QRS DURATION:** _____ (normal or too long). **Q-T INTERVAL:** _____ (normal, too long, or too short). **P′ WAVES:** _____ (present or absent). **JUNCTIONAL ECTOPIC BEATS:** _____ (present or absent).

Conclusion: _____

_____

ANALYSIS

RATE: 120/min. (tachycardia). RHYTHM: irregular and supraventricular. P-R INTERVAL: 0.13 sec. (normal). QRS DURATION: 0.08 sec. (normal). Q-T INTERVAL: 0.42 sec. (too long). P′ WAVES: present. JUNCTIONAL ECTOPIC BEATS: present.

Conclusion: This is a nonparoxysmal supraventricular (junctional) tachycardia. Usually this arrhythmia manifests with a rate of 70 to 130/min. and is commonly the result of digitalis excess. The slight irregularity in the tracing is the result of a reciprocal beat, sinus capture (second beat, P-R interval: 0.13 sec.) or another ectopic focus.

This arrhythmia is thought to be the result of enhanced automaticity in the A-V junction as opposed to the reentry mechanism seen in paroxysmal supraventricular tachycardia.

EXERCISE 3-6

V₁

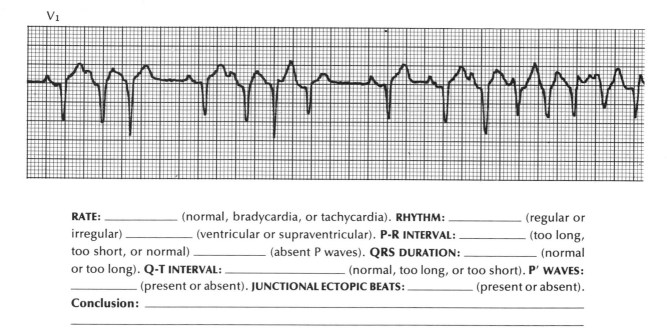

RATE: _____ (normal, bradycardia, or tachycardia). **RHYTHM:** _____ (regular or irregular) _____ (ventricular or supraventricular). **P-R INTERVAL:** _____ (too long, too short, or normal) _____ (absent P waves). **QRS DURATION:** _____ (normal or too long). **Q-T INTERVAL:** _____ (normal, too long, or too short). **P′ WAVES:** _____ (present or absent). **JUNCTIONAL ECTOPIC BEATS:** _____ (present or absent).

Conclusion: _____

_____

ANALYSIS

RATE: 100-155/min. (tachycardia). RHYTHM: irregular and supraventricular. P-R INTERVAL: 0.16 sec. (normal). QRS DURATION: 0.08 sec. (normal). Q-T INTERVAL: 0.26 sec. (too short). P′ WAVES: present. JUNCTIONAL ECTOPIC BEATS: absent.

Conclusion: This tracing shows bursts of PAT, which are the result of very early P′ waves. There are three sinus P waves—one at the beginning of the tracing, one after the first pause, and two following the second pause. There is some somatic tremor artifact, which is probably the cause of the distortion of the fourth P wave. The two P waves in a row (middle of the tracing) allow us to note that the underlying sinus rhythm is 100/min. This, along with the frequent PACs, should prompt a full physical assessment of the patient.

EXERCISE 3-7

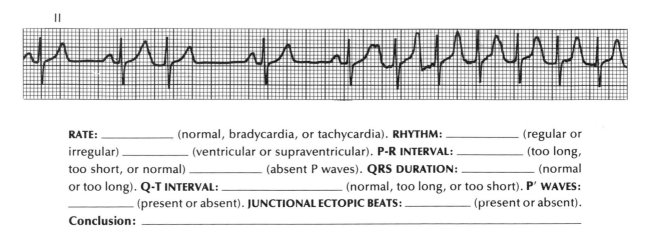

II

RATE: _____ (normal, bradycardia, or tachycardia). **RHYTHM:** _____ (regular or irregular) _____ (ventricular or supraventricular). **P-R INTERVAL:** _____ (too long, too short, or normal) _____ (absent P waves). **QRS DURATION:** _____ (normal or too long). **Q-T INTERVAL:** _____ (normal, too long, or too short). **P′ WAVES:** _____ (present or absent). **JUNCTIONAL ECTOPIC BEATS:** _____ (present or absent).

Conclusion: _____

_____

ANALYSIS

RATE: 70-140/min. (tachycardia). RHYTHM: irregular and supraventricular. P-R INTERVAL: 0.14 sec. (normal). QRS DURATION: 0.08 sec. (normal). Q-T INTERVAL: 0.32 sec. (too short). P′ WAVES: present. JUNCTIONAL ECTOPIC BEATS: absent.

Conclusion: There is a PAC in the second T wave causing it to be taller, more peaked, and broader than the preceding T wave. Two normal sinus beats and another P′ wave hiding in a T follow. This time a reciprocating mechanism is set up within the A-V junction, resulting in PAT. This mechanism is discussed in exercise 2-8.

EXERCISE 3-8

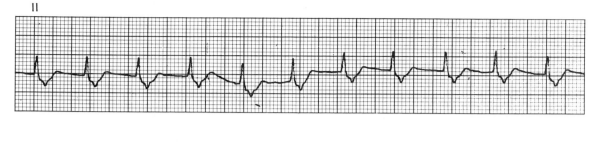

II

RATE: _____ (normal, bradycardia, or tachycardia). **RHYTHM:** _____ (regular or irregular) _____ (ventricular or supraventricular). **P-R INTERVAL:** _____ (too long, too short, or normal) _____ (absent P waves). **QRS DURATION:** _____ (normal or too long). **Q-T INTERVAL:** _____ (normal, too long, or too short). **P′ WAVES:** _____ (present or absent). **JUNCTIONAL ECTOPIC BEATS:** _____ (present or absent). **Conclusion:** _____

_____

ANALYSIS

RATE: 110/min. (tachycardia). RHYTHM: regular and supraventricular. P-R INTERVAL: absent P waves. QRS DURATION: 0.06 sec. (normal). Q-T INTERVAL: 0.28 sec. (normal). P′ WAVES: present. JUNCTIONAL ECTOPIC BEATS: present.

Conclusion: This tracing, as with exercise 3-5, is an example of nonparoxysmal junctional tachycardia. There are obviously no P waves in front of the ventricular complexes. Since the rhythm is absolutely regular and the ventricular complexes are normal, you can safely assume that this is a junctional rhythm (tachycardia). This is not an escape mechanism but, rather, active ectopy. If the junctional focus would slow down, the sinus node would probably regain control. In this junctional rhythm there happens to be retrograde conduction to the atria, as manifested by the negative P′ wave seen after each QRS complex (just at the peak of the inverted T wave). The position of the P′ wave relative to the QRS complex is a function of the speed of antegrade and retrograde conduction. The ventricles in this case are activated before the atria, causing the P′ wave to follow the QRS.

EXERCISE 3-9

V₁

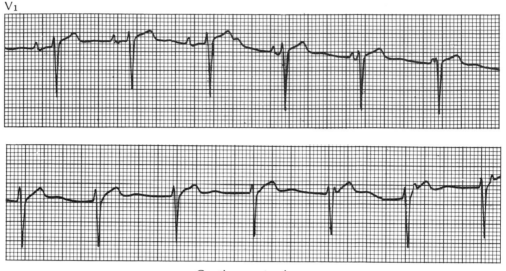

Continuous tracings.

RATE: _____ (normal, bradycardia, or tachycardia). **RHYTHM:** _____ (regular or irregular) _____ (ventricular or supraventricular). **P-R INTERVAL:** _____ (too long, too short, or normal) _____ (absent P waves). **QRS DURATION:** _____ (normal or too long). **Q-T INTERVAL:** _____ (normal, too long, or too short). **P′ WAVES:** _____ (present or absent). **JUNCTIONAL ECTOPIC BEATS:** _____ (present or absent).

Conclusion: _____

_____

ANALYSIS

RATE: 74/min. (normal). RHYTHM: regular and supraventricular. P-R INTERVAL: 0.20 sec. (normal; constant). QRS COMPLEX: 0.10 sec. (normal). Q-T INTERVAL: 0.32 sec. (too short). P′ WAVES: absent. JUNCTIONAL ECTOPIC BEATS: present.

Conclusion: This is a nonparoxysmal junctional tachycardia, resulting in A-V dissociation. The P waves can be seen getting closer and closer to the QRS complex until they are hidden within it. Then they emerge, looking like an R′ wave after the QRS. There is an underlying sinus arrhythmia, the sinus node slowing down from a rate of 74-70/min. This is certainly no cause for the A-V junction to take over at a rate of 73/min. The inherent rate of the A-V junction is 40-60/min.

EXERCISE 3-10

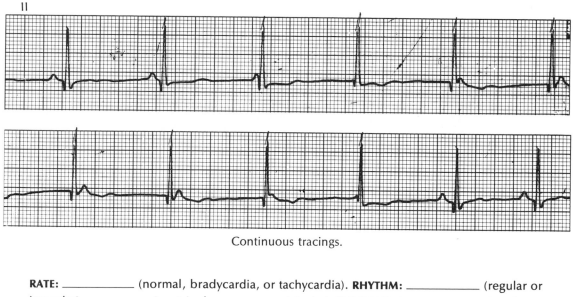

Continuous tracings.

RATE: _____ (normal, bradycardia, or tachycardia). **RHYTHM:** _____ (regular or irregular) _____ (ventricular or supraventricular). **P-R INTERVAL:** _____ (too long, too short, or normal) _____ (absent P waves). **QRS DURATION:** _____ (normal or too long). **Q-T INTERVAL:** _____ (normal, too long, or too short). **P' WAVES:** _____ (present or absent). **JUNCTIONAL ECTOPIC BEATS:** _____ (present or absent).

Conclusion: _____

_____

ANALYSIS

RATE: 58/min. (bradycardia). **RHYTHM:** regular and supraventricular. **P-R INTERVAL:** 0.16 sec. (normal). **QRS DURATION:** 0.10 sec. (normal). **Q-T INTERVAL:** difficult to determine. **P' WAVES:** absent. **VENTRICULAR ECTOPIC BEATS:** absent. **JUNCTIONAL ECTOPIC BEATS:** present.

Conclusion: This is a sinus bradycardia with a junctional escape rhythm. The result is A-V dissociation. The rate of the sinus node (58/min.) is the same as the inherent rate of the A-V junction. When the sinus node slows down enough, the pacemaker cells of the A-V junction discharge before they can be discharged by the impulse from the higher pacemaker (third beat). The junctional ectopic focus is in this case a protective mechanism rather than an active intrusion.

The term "A-V dissociation" should never be used by itself, since this condition may be the result of either enhanced automaticity of the junctional cells, as in exercise 3-9, or the junctional rhythm may simply be a normal, protective mechanism. The difference in clinical implications between the two makes the differential diagnosis important.

EXERCISE 3-11

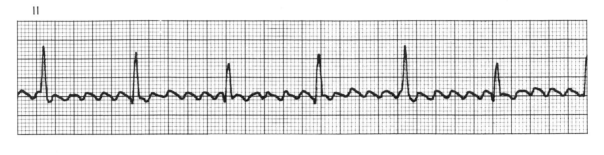

II

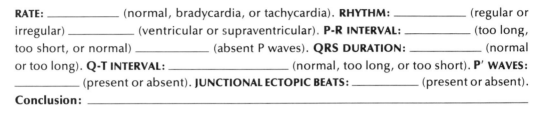

RATE: _____ (normal, bradycardia, or tachycardia). **RHYTHM:** _____ (regular or irregular) _____ (ventricular or supraventricular). **P-R INTERVAL:** _____ (too long, too short, or normal) _____ (absent P waves). **QRS DURATION:** _____ (normal or too long). **Q-T INTERVAL:** _____ (normal, too long, or too short). **P′ WAVES:** _____ (present or absent). **JUNCTIONAL ECTOPIC BEATS:** _____ (present or absent).

Conclusion: _____

_____

ANALYSIS

RATE: 62/min. (normal). RHYTHM: regular and supraventricular. P-R INTERVAL: absent P waves. QRS DURATION: 0.10 sec. (normal). Q-T INTERVAL: impossible to determine. P′ WAVES: present at a rate of 350/min. VENTRICULAR ECTOPIC BEATS: absent. JUNCTIONAL ECTOPIC BEATS: present.

Conclusion: The typical sawtooth pattern of atrial flutter is seen throughout the strip. However, there is no constant relationship between the flutter waves and the QRS complex. This is a sign of A-V dissociation or heart block coexisting with the atrial flutter. It is most probably A-V dissociation with capture, since the ventricular rhythm is not absolutely regular. This means that the atria are beating at a rate of 350/min. but that only an occasional impulse is being conducted to the ventricles, which are mainly under the control of an independent junctional focus with a rate of 62/min.

EXERCISE 3-12

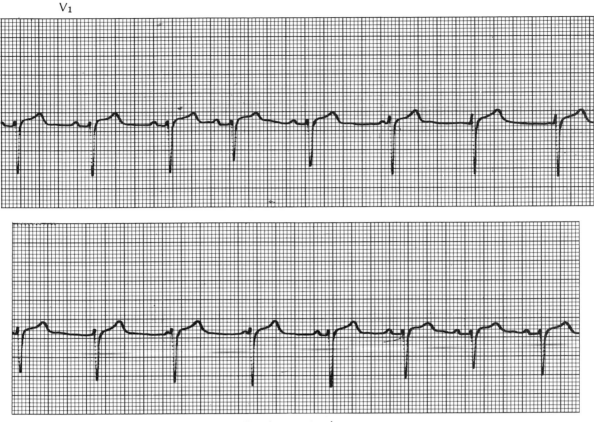

V₁

Continuous tracings.

RATE: _____ (normal, bradycardia, or tachycardia). **RHYTHM:** _____ (regular or irregular) _____ (ventricular or supraventricular). **P-R INTERVAL:** _____ (too long, too short, or normal) _____ (absent P waves). **QRS DURATION:** _____ (normal or too long). **Q-T INTERVAL:** _____ (normal, too long, or too short). **P′ WAVES:** _____ (present or absent). **JUNCTIONAL ECTOPIC BEATS:** _____ (present or absent).
Conclusion: _____

_____

ANALYSIS

RATE: 72-75/min. (normal). **RHYTHM:** irregular and supraventricular. **P-R INTERVAL:** 0.16 sec. (normal). **QRS DURATION:** 0.08 sec. (normal). **Q-T INTERVAL:** 0.36 sec. (normal). **P′ WAVES:** absent. **JUNCTIONAL ECTOPIC BEATS:** present.
Conclusion: This tracing is almost the same as the one in exercise 3-9. Were you able to make the diagnosis of nonparoxysmal junctional tachycardia as a cause of A-V dissociation? The rate of the sinus node is adequate at 75/min. and slows down to approximately 62/min. because of a sinus arrhythmia. At this time a junctional focus takes over at an enhanced rate of 68/min. (junctional tachycardia) and "warms up" to a rate of 72/min. before the sinus rhythm finally is fast enough to take over again at a heart rate of 80/min.

The problem is not that of sinus arrhythmia or A-V dissociation. Clearly the A-V junctional pacemaker should not be manifesting itself at an enhanced rate of 68-72/min. The possible causes of nonparoxysmal junctional tachycardia are digitalis toxicity, acute myocardial infarction, or acute rheumatic fever.[64-67]

EXERCISE 3-13

V₁

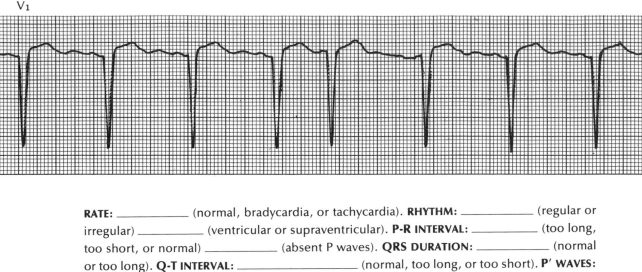

RATE: _____ (normal, bradycardia, or tachycardia). **RHYTHM:** _____ (regular or irregular) _____ (ventricular or supraventricular). **P-R INTERVAL:** _____ (too long, too short, or normal) _____ (absent P waves). **QRS DURATION:** _____ (normal or too long). **Q-T INTERVAL:** _____ (normal, too long, or too short). **P′ WAVES:** _____ (present or absent). **JUNCTIONAL ECTOPIC BEATS:** _____ (present or absent).

Conclusion: _____

_____

ANALYSIS

RATE: 65/min. (normal). **RHYTHM:** irregular and supraventricular. **P-R INTERVAL:** 0.16 sec. (normal). **QRS DURATION:** 0.10 sec. (normal). **Q-T INTERVAL:** 0.44 sec. (long). **P′ WAVES:** present. **JUNCTIONAL ECTOPIC BEATS:** present.

Conclusion: There is a single PJC in this tracing. It occurs coincidental with the U wave of the fourth complex. The presence of overdrive suppression (see exercise 2-5) or less than a full compensatory pause, as seen above, are evidence that the sinus node was depolarized prematurely by retrograde conduction from the junctional pacemaker. As mentioned before, whether or not this has occurred is clinically unimportant. However, an awareness of such a mechanism gives you more background in the understanding of electrocardiography and the comprehension of why you measure for a compensatory pause at all.

It is interesting to note that the P-R interval after the PJC is longer than the others. This is probably due to physiological refractoriness, which may have been caused by concealed antegrade reentry of the retrograde impulse back into the A-V node.

EXERCISE 3-14

II

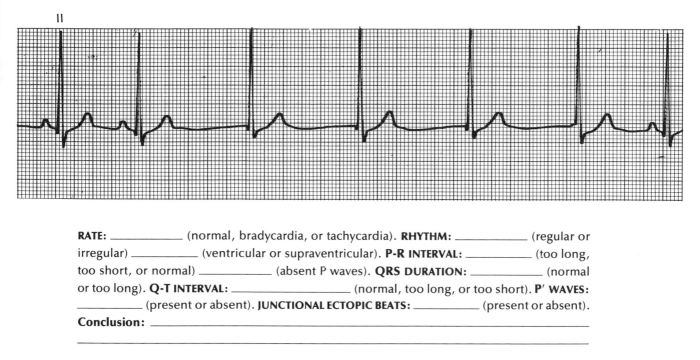

RATE: _____ (normal, bradycardia, or tachycardia). **RHYTHM:** _____ (regular or irregular) _____ (ventricular or supraventricular). **P-R INTERVAL:** _____ (too long, too short, or normal) _____ (absent P waves). **QRS DURATION:** _____ (normal or too long). **Q-T INTERVAL:** _____ (normal, too long, or too short). **P′ WAVES:** _____ (present or absent). **JUNCTIONAL ECTOPIC BEATS:** _____ (present or absent).

Conclusion: _____

_____

ANALYSIS

RATE: 52-60/min. (bradycardia). **RHYTHM:** irregular and supraventricular. **P-R INTERVAL:** 0.16 sec. (normal). **QRS DURATION:** 0.10 sec. (normal). **Q-T INTERVAL:** 0.40 sec. (normal). **P′ WAVES:** absent. **JUNCTIONAL ECTOPIC BEATS:** present.

Conclusion: Here is a junctional escape mechanism that is the result of an abrupt slowing or cessation of the sinus node impulse. When the sinus impulse fails to arrive at the A-V junction, these pacemaker cells protect the ventricles at a normal escape rate (in this case, 52/min.). In the fourth junctional escape beat (sixth complex) the sinus P wave can be seen distorting the q wave.

EXERCISE 3-15

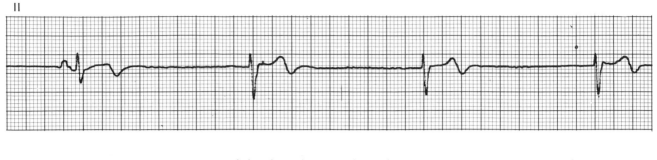

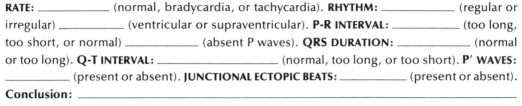

RATE: _____ (normal, bradycardia, or tachycardia). **RHYTHM:** _____ (regular or irregular) _____ (ventricular or supraventricular). **P-R INTERVAL:** _____ (too long, too short, or normal) _____ (absent P waves). **QRS DURATION:** _____ (normal or too long). **Q-T INTERVAL:** _____ (normal, too long, or too short). **P′ WAVES:** _____ (present or absent). **JUNCTIONAL ECTOPIC BEATS:** _____ (present or absent).

Conclusion: _____

_____

ANALYSIS

RATE: 33/min. (bradycardia). RHYTHM: irregular and supraventricular. P-R INTERVAL: 0.14 sec. (normal). QRS DURATION: 0.08-0.09 sec. (normal). Q-T INTERVAL: 0.52 sec. (normal). P′ WAVES: absent. JUNCTIONAL ECTOPIC BEATS: present.

Conclusion: The junctional escape rhythm in this tracing is the result of a profound sinus bradycardia and sinus arrhythmia. The first beat is sinus conducted. Note the different morphology between the junctional escape beat and the sinus conducted one (see exercise 3-3).[61,62] The hemodynamic impact of this profound bradycardia will determine the treatment. Atropine may be given or a pacemaker inserted (see p. 9).

EXERCISE 3-16

II

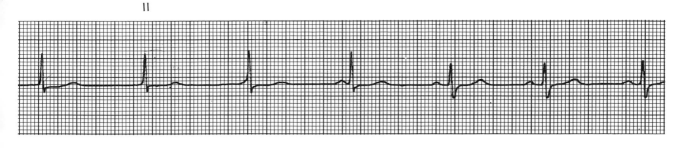

RATE: _____ (normal, bradycardia, or tachycardia). **RHYTHM:** _____ (regular or irregular) _____ (ventricular or supraventricular). **P-R INTERVAL:** _____ (too long, too short, or normal) _____ (absent P waves). **QRS DURATION:** _____ (normal or too long). **Q-T INTERVAL:** _____ (normal, too long, or too short). **P' WAVES:** _____ (present or absent). **JUNCTIONAL ECTOPIC BEATS:** _____ (present or absent).

Conclusion: _____

_____

ANALYSIS

RATE: 55-58/min. (bradycardia). **RHYTHM:** irregular and supraventricular. **P-R INTERVAL:** 0.16 sec. (normal). **QRS DURATION:** 0.08 sec. (normal). **Q-T INTERVAL:** 0.41 sec. (normal). **P' WAVES:** absent. **JUNCTIONAL ECTOPIC BEATS:** present.

Conclusion: The junctional escape mechanism seen in this tracing, as in the previous one, is the result of sinus arrhythmia and a sinus bradycardia. The inherent rate of this individual's A-V junctional pacemaker is 55/min. When the sinus rate slows down to less than that, the latent junctional pacemaker escapes and protects the ventricles at a slower pace. The sinus P wave can be seen speeding up and emerging from the third complex. By the fourth complex it is in front of the ventricular complex but not far enough in front to capture since this patient's P-R interval is 0.16 sec., and the junction fires before that time. The fifth complex is a sinus conducted beat.

The term "A-V dissociation" is generally used to describe this arrhythmia. It is an unfortunate term because it does not differentiate among nonparoxysmal junctional tachycardia, sinus bradycardia and junctional escape, sinus exit block and junctional escape, or the junctional escape that results from the bradycardia of second-degree heart block. I feel that the term A-V dissociation should be eliminated altogether, and the basic mechanism should simply be described, whether it is a junctional tachycardia or a particular arrhythmia resulting in junctional escape.

EXERCISE 3-17

II

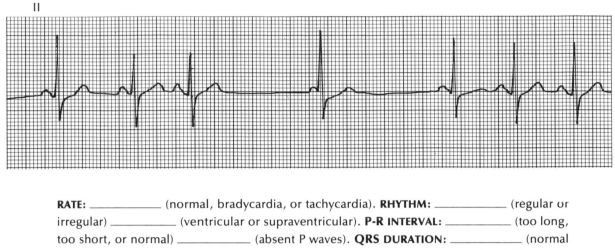

RATE: _____ (normal, bradycardia, or tachycardia). **RHYTHM:** _____ (regular or irregular) _____ (ventricular or supraventricular). **P-R INTERVAL:** _____ (too long, too short, or normal) _____ (absent P waves). **QRS DURATION:** _____ (normal or too long). **Q-T INTERVAL:** _____ (normal, too long, or too short). **P' WAVES:** _____ (present or absent). **JUNCTIONAL ECTOPIC BEATS:** _____ (present or absent).

Conclusion: _____

_____

ANALYSIS

RATE: 60-70/min. (normal). **RHYTHM:** irregular and supraventricular. **P-R INTERVAL:** 0.14 sec. (normal). **QRS DURATION:** 0.08 sec. (normal). **Q-T INTERVAL:** varies (normal). **P' WAVES:** present. **JUNCTIONAL ECTOPIC BEATS:** present.

Conclusion: There is a PAC and a junctional escape beat in this tracing. The third P wave is premature and has a different morphology from the two preceding sinus P waves. The next sinus P wave is delayed, perhaps due to a sinus arrhythmia or the effects of very marked overdrive suppression. There is a junctional escape beat before this P wave can conduct. The next sinus P wave is also delayed, after which the sinus rhythm increases to about 95/min. Note how the refractory period changes with the heart rate, as reflected in the changing Q-T intervals.

EXERCISE 3-18

V₁

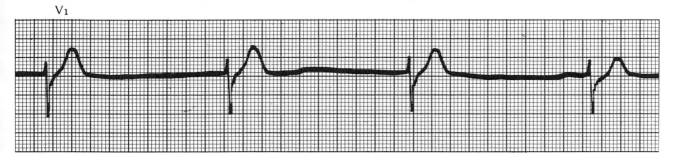

RATE: _____ (normal, bradycardia, or tachycardia). **RHYTHM:** _____ (regular or irregular) _____ (ventricular or supraventricular). **P-R INTERVAL:** _____ (too long, too short, or normal) _____ (absent P waves). **QRS DURATION:** _____ (normal or too long). **Q-T INTERVAL:** _____ (normal, too long, or too short). **P' WAVES:** _____ (present or absent). **JUNCTIONAL ECTOPIC BEATS:** _____ (present or absent).

Conclusion: _____

_____

ANALYSIS

RATE: 31/min. (bradycardia). **RHYTHM:** regular and supraventricular. **P-R INTERVAL:** absent P waves. **QRS DURATION:** 0.08 sec. (normal). **Q-T INTERVAL:** 0.44 sec. (normal). **P' WAVES:** not seen. **JUNCTIONAL ECTOPIC BEATS:** present.

Conclusion: This is a profound bradycardia and usually requires a pacemaker. In this particular lead there appears to be a junctional escape mechanism. There is no evidence of a P wave; however, you should search all of the other leads before deciding that there indeed are no P waves. There may or may not be retrograde activation of the atria during the QRS

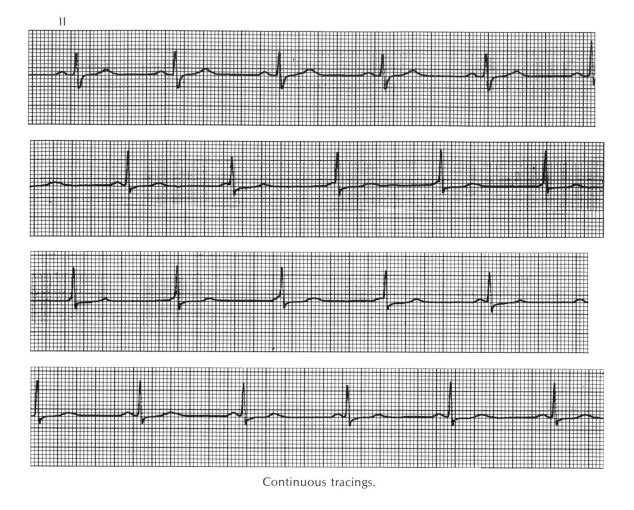

Continuous tracings.

RATE: _____ (normal, bradycardia, or tachycardia). **RHYTHM:** _____ (regular or irregular) _____ (ventricular or supraventricular). **P-R INTERVAL:** _____ (too long, too short, or normal) _____ (absent P waves). **QRS DURATION:** _____ (normal or too long). **Q-T INTERVAL:** _____ (normal, too long, or too short). **P′ WAVES:** _____ (present or absent). **JUNCTIONAL ECTOPIC BEATS:** _____ (present or absent).

Conclusion: _____

_____

ANALYSIS

RATE: 55/min. (bradycardia). RHYTHM: regular and supraventricular. P-R INTERVAL: 0.18 sec. (normal; constant). QRS DURATION: 0.09 sec. (normal). Q-T INTERVAL: 0.42 sec. (normal). P′ WAVES: absent. JUNCTIONAL ECTOPIC BEATS: present.

Conclusion: There is an underlying sinus bradycardia, with the sinus node beating at a rate of 55/min. and a junctional escape rhythm of 54/min. The onset of A-V dissociation can be seen in the first complex of the second strip. Because of the almost identical rates of the two pacemakers, an isorhythmic dissociation is maintained throughout the remainder of the tracing. The sinus-conducted beats are easy to distinguish from the junctional escape complexes because each has a different morphology, the former being conducted in 0.09 sec. with a deep s wave and the latter being conducted in 0.06 sec. with a small s wave. The P-R interval will also help you to determine when the sinus node is conducting. In this patient, it must reach 0.18 sec. before there can be capture. This occurs only in the first five complexes.

EXERCISE 3-20

V₁

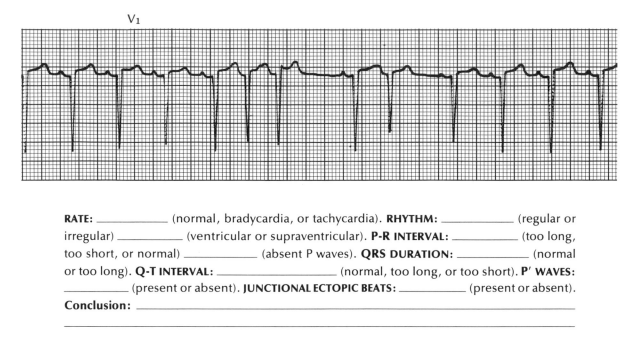

RATE: _____ (normal, bradycardia, or tachycardia). **RHYTHM:** _____ (regular or irregular) _____ (ventricular or supraventricular). **P-R INTERVAL:** _____ (too long, too short, or normal) _____ (absent P waves). **QRS DURATION:** _____ (normal or too long). **Q-T INTERVAL:** _____ (normal, too long, or too short). **P′ WAVES:** _____ (present or absent). **JUNCTIONAL ECTOPIC BEATS:** _____ (present or absent).

Conclusion: _____

_____

ANALYSIS

RATE: 120-150/min. (tachycardia). **RHYTHM:** irregular and supraventricular. **P-R INTERVAL:** 0.12 sec. (normal). **QRS DURATION:** 0.06 sec. (normal). **Q-T INTERVAL:** 0.28 sec. (normal). **P′ WAVES:** present. **JUNCTIONAL ECTOPIC BEATS:** absent.

Conclusion: The underlying rhythm here is a sinus tachycardia. There are PACs (sixth and ninth beats), the first of which is followed by a brief, reciprocating mechanism.

The combination of sinus tachycardia and frequent PACs should alert you to the possibility of congestive heart failure. The reciprocating mechanism briefly manifested here could be sustained and could produce a ventricular rate in excess of 200/min. This may cause an extension of the infarction. The underlying sinus tachycardia itself contributes to a decrease in cardiac output and coronary perfusion.

EXERCISE 3-21

II

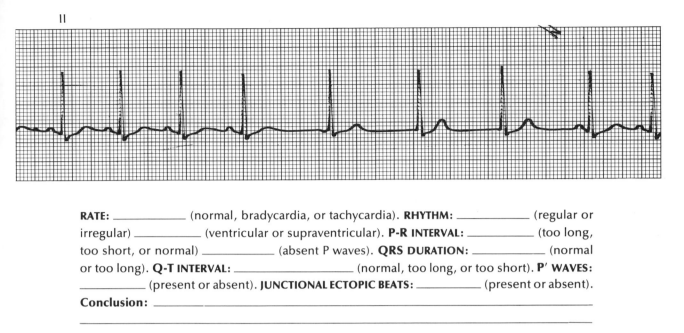

RATE: _____ (normal, bradycardia, or tachycardia). **RHYTHM:** _____ (regular or irregular) _____ (ventricular or supraventricular). **P-R INTERVAL:** _____ (too long, too short, or normal) _____ (absent P waves). **QRS DURATION:** _____ (normal or too long). **Q-T INTERVAL:** _____ (normal, too long, or too short). **P′ WAVES:** _____ (present or absent). **JUNCTIONAL ECTOPIC BEATS:** _____ (present or absent).

Conclusion: _____

_____

ANALYSIS

RATE: 65-90/min. (normal). RHYTHM: irregular and supraventricular. P-R INTERVAL: 0.14 sec. (normal). QRS DURATION: 0.09 sec. (normal). Q-T INTERVAL: varies (normal). P′ WAVES: absent. JUNCTIONAL ECTOPIC BEATS: present and escape.

Conclusion: This is a rather marked sinus arrhythmia resulting in junctional escape beats. At the end of the tracing the P waves finally increase enough in rate to capture. It is, however, only the last P wave that conducts. The preceding P wave does not conduct, since the P-R interval is shorter than the ones that are known to conduct and the ventricular beat is right on time with the preceding escape junctional rhythm.

EXERCISE 3-22

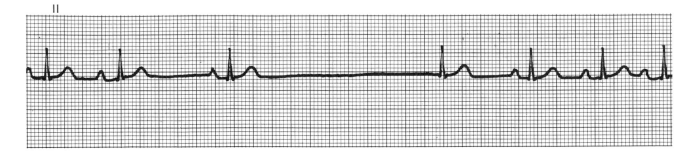

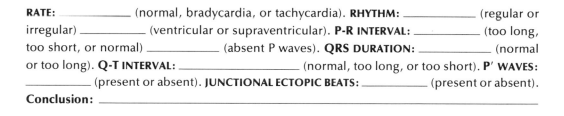

RATE: _____ (normal, bradycardia, or tachycardia). **RHYTHM:** _____ (regular or irregular) _____ (ventricular or supraventricular). **P-R INTERVAL:** _____ (too long, too short, or normal) _____ (absent P waves). **QRS DURATION:** _____ (normal or too long). **Q-T INTERVAL:** _____ (normal, too long, or too short). **P' WAVES:** _____ (present or absent). **JUNCTIONAL ECTOPIC BEATS:** _____ (present or absent).

Conclusion: _____

_____

ANALYSIS

RATE: 60-90/min. (normal). **RHYTHM:** irregular and supraventricular. **P-R INTERVAL:** varies. **QRS DURATION:** 0.10 sec. (normal). **Q-T INTERVAL:** varies (normal). **P' WAVES:** present. **JUNCTIONAL ECTOPIC BEATS:** present.

Conclusion: This tracing reflects sinus exit block and also qualifies as a sick sinus syndrome, since the sinus rate after the long pause jumps to 90/min. There is an atrial escape beat, a junctional escape beat, and an underlying second-degree heart block (Wenckebach). The latter condition is covered in Chapter 5.

There are two normal sinus beats at the beginning of the tracing, followed by a period of sinus inactivity. This is terminated by the atrial escape beat (the third P wave). It is of different morphology from the sinus P waves and demonstrates the latent pacemaker function of the atrial specialized conductive system. Another period of sinus exit block ensues. This time it is terminated by a junctional escape beat.

The hemodynamic effects of such long pauses in rhythm can be very profound and damaging. Patients with sick sinus syndrome may not respond favorably to atropine and may require a pacemaker.

EXERCISE 3-23

V₁

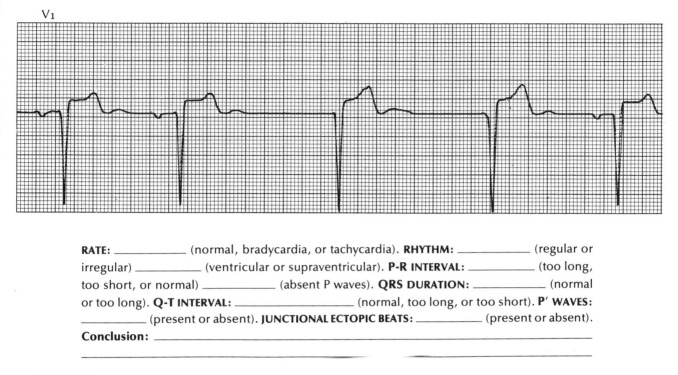

RATE: _____ (normal, bradycardia, or tachycardia). **RHYTHM:** _____ (regular or irregular) _____ (ventricular or supraventricular). **P-R INTERVAL:** _____ (too long, too short, or normal) _____ (absent P waves). **QRS DURATION:** _____ (normal or too long). **Q-T INTERVAL:** _____ (normal, too long, or too short). **P' WAVES:** _____ (present or absent). **JUNCTIONAL ECTOPIC BEATS:** _____ (present or absent).

Conclusion: _____

_____

ANALYSIS

RATE: 35-40/min. (bradycardia). RHYTHM: irregular and supraventricular. P-R INTERVAL: 0.20 sec. (normal). QRS DURATION: 0.10 sec. (normal). Q-T INTERVAL: varies (normal). P' WAVES: absent. JUNCTIONAL ECTOPIC BEATS: present.

Conclusion: This is a sinus bradycardia and sinus arrhythmia with two junctional escape beats. There are probably sinus P waves in the T waves of the junctional beats. Remember that in V₁ the P wave may normally be positive, negative, or biphasic.

EXERCISE 3-24

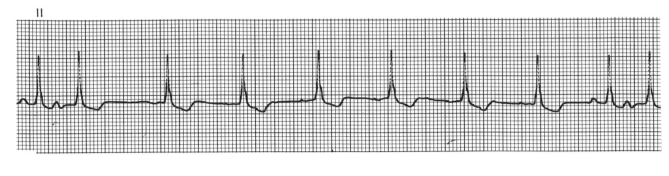

RATE: _____ (normal, bradycardia, or tachycardia). **RHYTHM:** _____ (regular or irregular) _____ (ventricular or supraventricular). **P-R INTERVAL:** _____ (too long, too short, or normal) _____ (absent P waves). **QRS DURATION:** _____ (normal or too long). **Q-T INTERVAL:** _____ (normal, too long, or too short). **P′ WAVES:** _____ (present or absent). **JUNCTIONAL ECTOPIC BEATS:** _____ (present or absent).

Conclusion: _____

_____

ANALYSIS

RATE: 75-80/min. (normal). **RHYTHM:** irregular and supraventricular. **P-R INTERVAL:** 0.16 sec. (normal). **QRS DURATION:** 0.08 sec. (normal). **Q-T INTERVAL:** varies (normal). **P′ WAVES:** present. **JUNCTIONAL ECTOPIC BEATS:** present.

Conclusion: In this tracing sinus P waves coupled with very early PACs are seen at the beginning and end of the strip. Evidently the PAC suppresses the sinus node enough to unmask a very active junctional ectopic focus. At first glance the rhythm after the first PAC looks like an escape mechanism. However, a rate of 75/min. is too fast for a passive escape response. This arrhythmia may be the result of digitalis toxicity.

EXERCISE 3-25

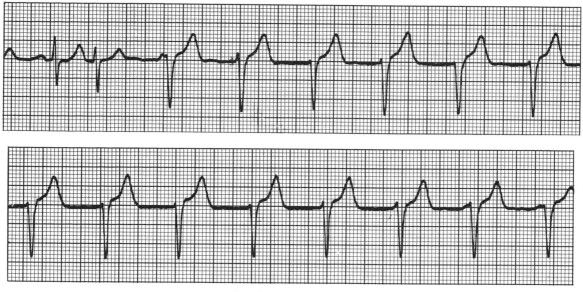

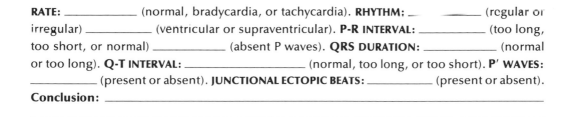

Continuous tracings.

RATE: _____ (normal, bradycardia, or tachycardia). **RHYTHM:** _____ (regular or irregular) _____ (ventricular or supraventricular). **P-R INTERVAL:** _____ (too long, too short, or normal) _____ (absent P waves). **QRS DURATION:** _____ (normal or too long). **Q-T INTERVAL:** _____ (normal, too long, or too short). **P′ WAVES:** _____ (present or absent). **JUNCTIONAL ECTOPIC BEATS:** _____ (present or absent).
Conclusion: _____
_____

ANALYSIS

RATE: 75-80/min. (normal). RHYTHM: irregular and supraventricular. **P-R** INTERVAL: 0.16 sec. (normal). **QRS DURATION:** 0.08 sec. (normal). **Q-T INTERVAL:** 0.36 sec. (normal). **P′ WAVES:** present. JUNCTIONAL ECTOPIC BEATS: present.
Conclusion: This tracing is almost like the previous one. There is one PAC that gives way to a nonparoxysmal junctional tachycardia with a rate of 75/min. The resulting A-V dissociation is easily seen as the P wave enters the junctional ectopic beat and then, in the second tracing, begins to emerge from it, looking like a wide r wave (fifth and sixth beats, second tracing).

CHAPTER 4
VENTRICULAR ECTOPICS

Beginning with this chapter the format for the evaluation of each rhythm strip includes the recognition of ventricular ectopic beats. This recognition is one of the most important ones you will make. It is the ventricular ectopics that threaten life. Immediately following myocardial infarction, ventricular ectopic activity can appear in the form of single premature ventricular contractions (PVCs), paroxysms of ventricular tachycardia, and ventricular fibrillation. It has been suggested by investigators that both reentry and enhanced automaticity play a role in the genesis of the arrhythmias in the acute stage of myocardial infarction.[70,71] During the chronic phase when anatomic and electrophysiological changes are stabilizing, reentry is thought to be the most likely mechanism. Several days or weeks after the acute myocardial infarction, long-lasting, stable episodes of ventricular tachycardia may occur. Such arrhythmias are thought to be due to enhanced automaticity and can be extremely resistant to drug therapy.

The reentry mechanism discussed relative to ventricular ectopics takes place within the His-Purkinje system. Ventricular reentry presupposes an area of decremental conduction and one-way block. If the pathway of decreased conduction velocity is long enough, the healthy myocardium will be nonrefractory by the time the impulse traverses the diseased tissue. Recapture of the healthy myocardium may then occur, and a reentry circuit is established as long as this one area of myocardium is out of phase with the rest of the ventricular tissue.

Your recognition of the PVC should include an assessment of how many forms the PVCs assume, how often they occur, from which ventricle, and how close to the T wave they are. PVCs occurring more than 5/min., emanating from the left ventricle, assuming more than one morphology, coinciding with or very close to the T wave, or appearing in pairs are all known to have more ominous implications and require more aggressive therapy than does the occasional, unifocal PVC.

EXERCISE 4-1

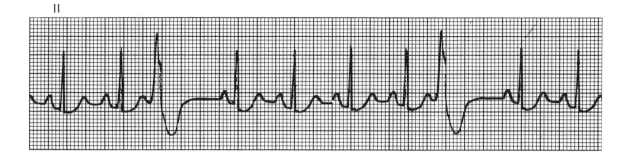

II

RATE: _____ (normal, bradycardia, or tachycardia). **RHYTHM:** _____ (regular or irregular) _____ (ventricular or supraventricular). **P-R INTERVAL:** _____ (too long, too short, or normal) _____ (absent P waves). **QRS DURATION:** _____ (normal or too long). **Q-T INTERVAL:** _____ (normal, too long, or too short). **P' WAVES:** _____ (present or absent). **JUNCTIONAL ECTOPIC BEATS:** _____ (present or absent).
VENTRICULAR ECTOPIC BEATS: _____ (present or absent) _____ (unifocal or multifocal) _____ (frequent or infrequent) _____ (R on T).
Conclusion: _____
_____

ANALYSIS

RATE: 100/min. (normal). RHYTHM: basically regular and supraventricular. P-R INTER-VAL: 0.16 sec. (normal; constant). QRS DURATION: 0.07 sec. (normal). Q-T INTERVAL: 0.32 sec. (normal). P' WAVES: absent. JUNCTIONAL ECTOPIC BEATS: absent. VENTRICULAR ECTOPIC BEATS: present, premature, frequent, and unifocal.

Conclusion: You probably had no difficulty in recognizing the two premature ven-tircular ectopic beats in this tracing. They have all the classic signs of the PVC. There is no related P wave, and they are broad and distorted, with an increased amplitude and a T wave of opposite polarity. Perhaps you also noticed that both PVCs are exactly coupled, or linked, to the preceding complex. In other words, the coupling interval between the R wave of the PVC and the R wave of the preceding complex is 0.36 sec. The interval is exactly the same in both instances, as if the PVC were somehow dependent on the preceding beat for its own generation. It is thought that exact coupling demonstrates a ventricular reentry mechanism. In such a case the sinus-conducted impulse would take the same time each beat to travel through the area of decreased conduction velocity and emerge to recapture the ventricles.

This mechanism presupposes (1) a one-way block, (2) an area of myocardium in which conduction velocity is slower than it is in the rest of the ventricle, and (3) a long enough pathway so that by the time the decelerated current emerges into healthy tissue, that tissue has already become nonrefractory and is ready to accept another impulse.

EXERCISE 4-2

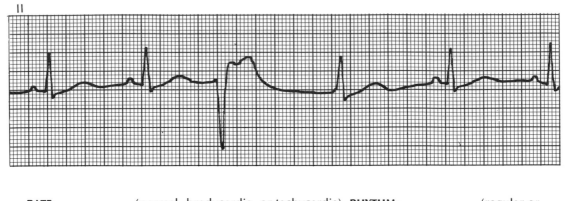

RATE: _____ (normal, bradycardia, or tachycardia). **RHYTHM:** _____ (regular or irregular) _____ (ventricular or supraventricular). **P-R INTERVAL:** _____ (too long, too short, or normal) _____ (absent P waves). **QRS DURATION:** _____ (normal or too long). **Q-T INTERVAL:** _____ (normal, too long, or too short). **P' WAVES:** _____ (present or absent). **JUNCTIONAL ECTOPIC BEATS:** _____ (present or absent). **VENTRICULAR ECTOPIC BEATS:** _____ (present or absent) _____ (unifocal or multifocal) _____ (frequent or infrequent) _____ (R on T). **Conclusion:** _____

ANALYSIS

RATE: 55-60/min. (bradycardia). **RHYTHM:** irregular and supraventricular with ventricular. **P-R INTERVAL:** 0.15 sec. (normal). **QRS DURATION:** 0.12 sec. (too long). **Q-T INTERVAL:** 0.52 sec. (too long). **P' WAVES:** absent. **JUNCTIONAL ECTOPIC BEATS:** present and escape. **VENTRICULAR ECTOPIC BEATS:** present.

Conclusion: There is one PVC in this tracing. Because the underlying rhythm is slow, the compensatory pause after the PVC allows for a junctional escape beat. In this complex the sinus P wave can be seen causing an initial slur in the QRS and making it look broader than it actually is.

The main concern here is, of course, the ventricular ectopic beat and not the junctional escape beat. The treatment of this arrhythmia would depend on the clinical picture and how many PVCs are occurring each minute. The bradycardia would not be treated unless the blood pressure was low or unless the PVCs were excessive and it was felt that an increase in sinus rate would suppress them.

EXERCISE 4-3

MCL₁

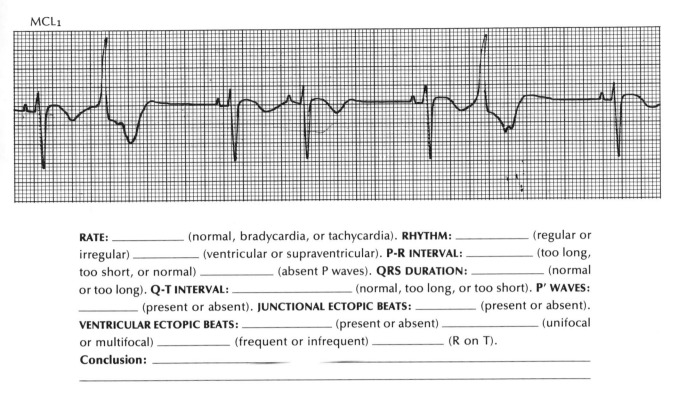

RATE: _____ (normal, bradycardia, or tachycardia). **RHYTHM:** _____ (regular or irregular) _____ (ventricular or supraventricular). **P-R INTERVAL:** _____ (too long, too short, or normal) _____ (absent P waves). **QRS DURATION:** _____ (normal or too long). **Q-T INTERVAL:** _____ (normal, too long, or too short). **P' WAVES:** _____ (present or absent). **JUNCTIONAL ECTOPIC BEATS:** _____ (present or absent). **VENTRICULAR ECTOPIC BEATS:** _____ (present or absent) _____ (unifocal or multifocal) _____ (frequent or infrequent) _____ (R on T). **Conclusion:** _____

ANALYSIS

RATE: 60-70/min. (normal). RHYTHM: irregular and supraventricular with ventricular. P-R INTERVAL: 0.12 sec. (normal). QRS DURATION: 0.11 sec. (too long). Q-T INTERVAL: 0.60 sec. (too long). P' WAVES: present. JUNCTIONAL ECTOPIC BEATS: absent. VENTRICULAR ECTOPIC BEATS: present and unifocal.

Conclusion: There are atrial and ventricular ectopies in this tracing. The PVCs are the second and sixth beats. The normal sinus P waves can be seen right on time in the T waves of the PVCs. The fourth beat is a PAC. Frequent PVCs are usually treated with lidocaine.

EXERCISE 4-4

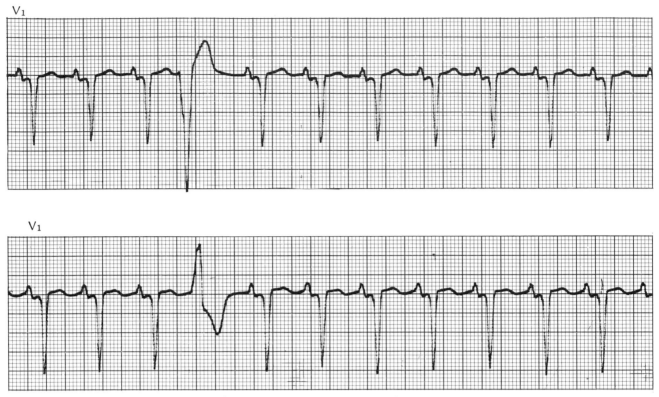

Same patient. Tracings not continuous.

RATE: _____ (normal, bradycardia, or tachycardia). **RHYTHM:** _____ (regular or irregular) _____ (ventricular or supraventricular). **P-R INTERVAL:** _____ (too long, too short, or normal) _____ (absent P waves). **QRS DURATION:** _____ (normal or too long). **Q-T INTERVAL:** _____ (normal, too long, or too short). **P' WAVES:** _____ (present or absent). **JUNCTIONAL ECTOPIC BEATS:** _____ (present or absent). **VENTRICULAR ECTOPIC BEATS:** _____ (present or absent) _____ (unifocal or multifocal) _____ (frequent or infrequent) _____ (R on T). **Conclusion:** _____ _____

ANALYSIS

RATE: 98-100/min. (normal). RHYTHM: irregular and supraventricular with ventricular. P-R INTERVAL: 0.14 sec. (normal). QRS DURATION: 0.08 sec. (normal). Q-T INTERVAL: 0.29 sec. (normal). P' WAVES: absent. JUNCTIONAL ECTOPIC BEATS: absent. VENTRICULAR ECTOPIC BEATS: present and multifocal.

Conclusion: This patient is having both right and left ventricular PVCs. It is felt that the left ventricular PVC is more threatening than a PVC from the right ventricle because its location places it closer to the preceding refractory period.

The site of the ventricular ectopic focus is determined by observing the polarity of the ectopic complex in V_1. If the ectopic current originates in the right ventricle, it will proceed to the left and posteriorly, away from the positive electrode of V_1. A negative complex will then be inscribed. Conversely, if the ectopic current originates in the left ventricle, it will proceed toward the positive electrode of V_1. A positive complex will be inscribed.

It is also important to understand what a compensatory pause is and how you should use it as a diagnostic aid. In the preceding tracings, the P waves can be walked out right through the strip. The two PVCs do not interfere with the normal sinus rhythm. There is a pause because the P wave after the PVCs (in this case the P wave is buried in the ectopic T wave) is not conducted due to physiological refractoriness. However, in Chapters 2 and 3 we learned about overdrive suppression, in which case a PAC may suppress the sinus node, delaying the next P wave instead of causing it to come earlier as expected. Thus, a PAC can exactly simulate the uninterrupted sinus rhythm that accompanies a PVC. It is apparent then that the presence of a full compensatory pause can mean *either* atrial *or* ventricular ectopy. What then is the value of measuring it at all? When the compensatory pauses following an ectopic-looking beat is *less than full*, it is obvious that atrial ectopy is involved and that the sinus node has been "reset." The figure below illustrates this point. If you walk out the P waves through the tracing, you will find that there is less than a full compensatory pause after the broad premature beat. This tells of atrial involvement and will alert you to examine the T wave preceding the broad beat very carefully. It is different in shape than the other T waves and contains a P′ wave that is conducted with aberrancy. This is discussed in Chapter 7. Except for the fact that there is not a full compensatory pause, it exactly simulates a PVC. Remember then that the full compensatory pause proves nothing. It is only when the compensatory pause is less than full that the measurement is a diagnostic aid.

II

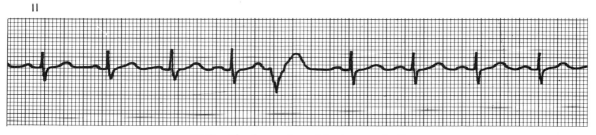
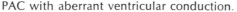

PAC with aberrant ventricular conduction.

EXERCISE 4-5

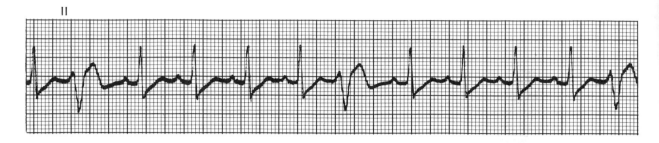

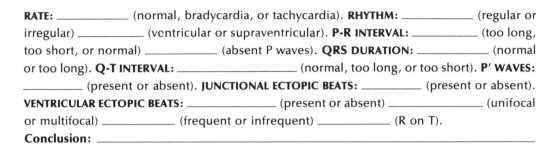

RATE: _____ (normal, bradycardia, or tachycardia). **RHYTHM:** _____ (regular or irregular) _____ (ventricular or supraventricular). **P-R INTERVAL:** _____ (too long, too short, or normal) _____ (absent P waves). **QRS DURATION:** _____ (normal or too long). **Q-T INTERVAL:** _____ (normal, too long, or too short). **P' WAVES:** _____ (present or absent). **JUNCTIONAL ECTOPIC BEATS:** _____ (present or absent). **VENTRICULAR ECTOPIC BEATS:** _____ (present or absent) _____ (unifocal or multifocal) _____ (frequent or infrequent) _____ (R on T). **Conclusion:** _____

ANALYSIS

RATE: 105/min. (tachycardia). **RHYTHM:** irregular and supraventricular with ventricular. **P-R INTERVAL:** 0.15 sec. (normal). **QRS DURATION:** 0.09 sec. (normal). **Q-T INTERVAL:** 0.31 sec. (normal). **P' WAVES:** absent. **JUNCTIONAL ECTOPIC BEATS:** absent. **VENTRICULAR ECTOPIC BEATS:** present, frequent, and unifocal.

Conclusion: In spite of an underlying AC interference throughout the tracing, three unifocal PVCs are easily seen. The accompanying sinus tachycardia may be attributed to one of a number of causes (such as fever, emotions, or physical activity). It may also be the response of the sinus node to a failing left ventricle. A thorough physical assessment should be carried out along with aggressive treatment of the ventricular ectopics.

EXERCISE 4-6

V₁

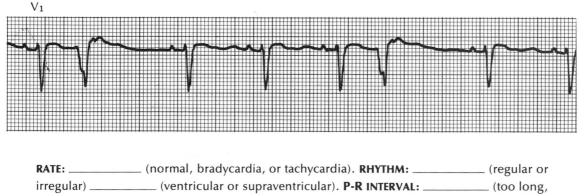

RATE: _____ (normal, bradycardia, or tachycardia). **RHYTHM:** _____ (regular or irregular) _____ (ventricular or supraventricular). **P-R INTERVAL:** _____ (too long, too short, or normal) _____ (absent P waves). **QRS DURATION:** _____ (normal or too long). **Q-T INTERVAL:** _____ (normal, too long, or too short). **P' WAVES:** _____ (present or absent). **JUNCTIONAL ECTOPIC BEATS:** _____ (present or absent).
VENTRICULAR ECTOPIC BEATS: _____ (present or absent) _____ (unifocal or multifocal) _____ (frequent or infrequent) _____ (R on T).
Conclusion: _____
_____

ANALYSIS

RATE: 73-75/min. (normal). **RHYTHM:** irregular and supraventricular with ventricular. **P-R INTERVAL:** 0.14 sec. (normal). **QRS DURATION:** 0.10 sec. (normal). **Q-T INTERVAL:** 0.28 sec. (normal). **P' WAVES:** present. **JUNCTIONAL ECTOPIC BEATS:** absent. **VENTRICULAR ECTOPIC BEATS:** present, unifocal, and frequent.

Conclusion: The two PVCs in this tracing have retrograde conduction to the atria. This means that the ventricular ectopic current traveled backward up the A-V junction to prematurely invade the atria. This will affect the sinus node just as any atrial ectopic stimulus would. The sinus node will either reset itself, causing the next expected sinus P wave to be earlier, or the P' wave will cause overdrive suppression, causing a delay in the next sinus discharge.

When you walk out the P waves, you will see that there is less than a full compensatory pause. Here is yet another cause for the compensatory pause to be less than full—retrograde conduction to the atria from a PVC. Therefore, when the sinus P wave after an anomalous-looking beat is found to be early (less than full compensatory pause), you are obliged to search not only the T wave preceding the beat in question but also the T wave following such a complex.

EXERCISE 4-7

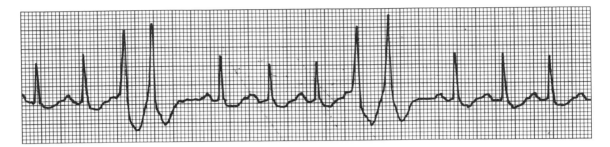

RATE: _____ (normal, bradycardia, or tachycardia). **RHYTHM:** _____ (regular or irregular) _____ (ventricular or supraventricular). **P-R INTERVAL:** _____ (too long, too short, or normal) _____ (absent P waves). **QRS DURATION:** _____ (normal or too long). **Q-T INTERVAL:** _____ (normal, too long, or too short). **P′ WAVES:** _____ (present or absent). **JUNCTIONAL ECTOPIC BEATS:** _____ (present or absent). **VENTRICULAR ECTOPIC BEATS:** _____ (present or absent) _____ (unifocal or multifocal) _____ (frequent or infrequent) _____ (R on T).

Conclusion: _____
_____

ANALYSIS

RATE: 110-120/min. (tachycardia). RHYTHM: irregular, supraventricular, and ventricular. P-R INTERVAL: 0.18 sec. (normal; constant). QRS DURATION: 0.08 sec. (normal). Q-T INTERVAL: difficult to determine. P′ WAVES: absent. JUNCTIONAL ECTOPIC BEATS: absent. VENTRICULAR ECTOPIC BEATS: present, premature, unifocal, and frequent.

Conclusion: The underlying rhythm is a sinus tachycardia, with somatic tremor slightly distorting the S-T segments and P waves. There are frequent PVCs (occurring in pairs or "back to back"), which certainly deserve prompt, aggressive treatment. When PVCs follow one another at a rapid rate, each succeeding ectopic beat depolarizes at a lower resting membrane potential, which causes dissimilar refractory periods and sets the ventricles up for fibrillation.

EXERCISE 4-8

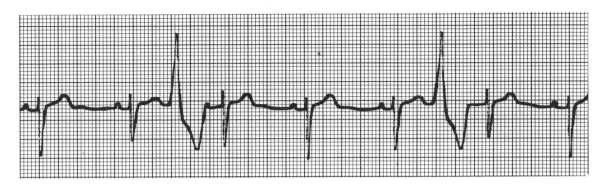

RATE: _____ (normal, bradycardia, or tachycardia). **RHYTHM:** _____ (regular or irregular) _____ (ventricular or supraventricular). **P-R INTERVAL:** _____ (too long, too short, or normal) _____ (absent P waves). **QRS DURATION:** _____ (normal or too long). **Q-T INTERVAL:** _____ (normal, too long, or too short). **P' WAVES:** _____ (present or absent). **JUNCTIONAL ECTOPIC BEATS:** _____ (present or absent). **VENTRICULAR ECTOPIC BEATS:** _____ (present or absent) _____ (unifocal or multifocal) _____ (frequent or infrequent) _____ (R on T).
Conclusion: _____

ANALYSIS

RATE: 90/min. (normal). **RHYTHM:** irregular and supraventricular with ventricular. **P-R INTERVAL:** 0.14 sec. (normal). **QRS DURATION:** 0.08 sec. (normal). **Q-T INTERVAL:** 0.36 sec. (short). **P' WAVES:** absent. **JUNCTIONAL ECTOPIC BEATS:** absent. **VENTRICULAR ECTOPIC BEATS:** present, unifocal, and frequent.

Conclusion: By now you will easily recognize ventricular ectopy. The PVCs in this tracing are called interpolated because they are sandwiched in between two normal sinus beats without disturbing the rhythm. The interpolated PVC is seen more often in a bradycardia than it is when the underlying rate approaches 70/min., as it does in this tracing.

The changing height of the sinus-conducted ventricular complexes is due to respirations.

EXERCISE 4-9

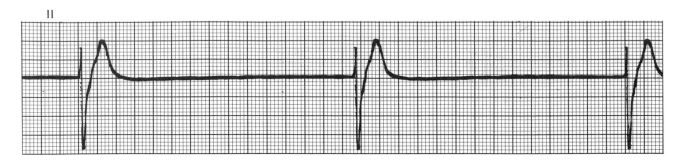

RATE: _____ (normal, bradycardia, or tachycardia). **RHYTHM:** _____ (regular or irregular) _____ (ventricular or supraventricular). **P-R INTERVAL:** _____ (too long, too short, or normal) _____ (absent P waves). **QRS DURATION:** _____ (normal or too long). **Q-T INTERVAL:** _____ (normal, too long, or too short). **P' WAVES:** _____ (present or absent). **JUNCTIONAL ECTOPIC BEATS:** _____ (present or absent). **VENTRICULAR ECTOPIC BEATS:** _____ (present or absent) _____ (unifocal or multifocal) _____ (frequent or infrequent) _____ (R on T). **Conclusion:** _____

_____

ANALYSIS

RATE: 20/min. (bradycardia). **RHYTHM:** regular and ventricular. **P-R INTERVAL:** absent P waves. **QRS DURATION:** 0.12 sec. (too long). **Q-T INTERVAL:** 0.36 sec. (too short). **P' WAVES:** absent. **JUNCTIONAL ECTOPIC BEATS:** absent. **VENTRICULAR ECTOPIC BEATS:** present (escape). **Conclusion:** This tracing represents a very slow idioventricular escape rhythm. No P waves are seen, although another lead might show some. Such a rhythm indicates that all pacemakers above this ventricular focus have failed.

EXERCISE 4-10

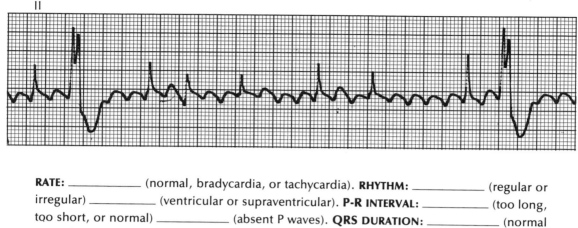

RATE: _____ (normal, bradycardia, or tachycardia). **RHYTHM:** _____ (regular or irregular) _____ (ventricular or supraventricular). **P-R INTERVAL:** _____ (too long, too short, or normal) _____ (absent P waves). **QRS DURATION:** _____ (normal or too long). **Q-T INTERVAL:** _____ (normal, too long, or too short). **P' WAVES:** _____ (present or absent). **JUNCTIONAL ECTOPIC BEATS:** _____ (present or absent). **VENTRICULAR ECTOPIC BEATS:** _____ (present or absent) _____ (unifocal or multifocal) _____ (frequent or infrequent) _____ (R on T). **Conclusion:** _____

_____

ANALYSIS

RATE: 90-100/min. (normal). **RHYTHM:** irregular and supraventricular with ventricular. **P-R INTERVAL:** absent P waves. **QRS DURATION:** 0.08 sec. (normal). **Q-T INTERVAL:** impossible to determine. **P' WAVES:** present and premature. **JUNCTIONAL ECTOPIC BEATS:** absent. **VENTRICULAR ECTOPIC BEATS:** present, unifocal, and frequent.

Conclusion: The distinctive sawtooth pattern of atrial flutter is unmistakable in this tracing. There is a variable conduction ratio, sometimes 2:1, 3:1, 4:1 and 5:1. The broad, distorted, ventricular complexes toward the beginning and end of the tracing are probably PVCs.

There is a differential diagnosis between ventricular ectopy and aberration. The principles governing the morphological distinction between the two are discussed in Chapter 8.

EXERCISE 4-11

II

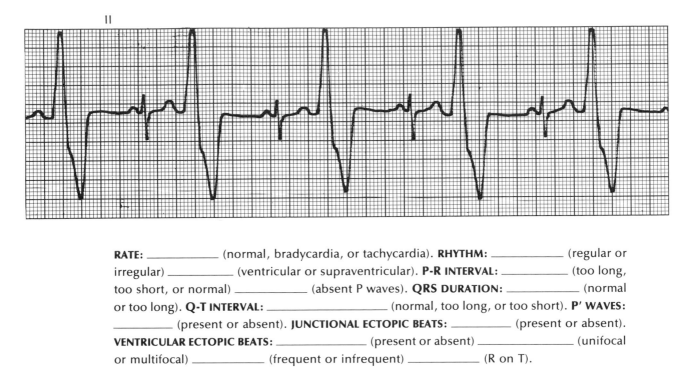

RATE: _____ (normal, bradycardia, or tachycardia). **RHYTHM:** _____ (regular or irregular) _____ (ventricular or supraventricular). **P-R INTERVAL:** _____ (too long, too short, or normal) _____ (absent P waves). **QRS DURATION:** _____ (normal or too long). **Q-T INTERVAL:** _____ (normal, too long, or too short). **P' WAVES:** _____ (present or absent). **JUNCTIONAL ECTOPIC BEATS:** _____ (present or absent). **VENTRICULAR ECTOPIC BEATS:** _____ (present or absent) _____ (unifocal or multifocal) _____ (frequent or infrequent) _____ (R on T). **Conclusion:** _____

ANALYSIS

RATE: 85/min. (normal). **RHYTHM:** irregular and bigeminal ventricular. **P-R INTERVAL:** 0.13 sec. (normal). **QRS DURATION:** 0.09 sec. (normal). **Q-T INTERVAL:** 0.41 sec. (normal). **P' WAVES:** absent. **JUNCTIONAL ECTOPIC BEATS:** absent. **VENTRICULAR ECTOPIC BEATS:** present, unifocal, and frequent.

Conclusion: When PVCs occur every other beat, as in this tracing, the term "bigeminy" is applied. This tracing gives you an opportunity to note the fixed coupling interval. If you measure the distance between a normally conducted ventricular complex and the PVC that follows it, you will find that the same distance links every other couplet in the tracing. This mechanism was explained in exercise 4-1.

V₁

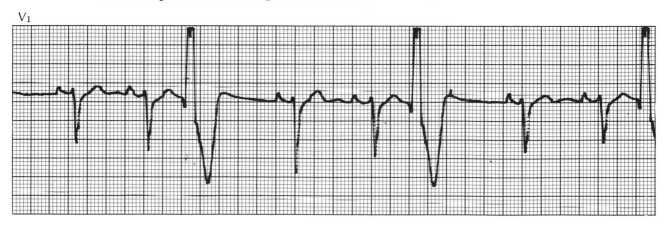

The above figure is an example of trigeminy. There is a PVC every third beat. Both arrhythmias are sometimes seen with digitalis toxicity but may be seen in patients with no symptoms of heart disease.

EXERCISE 4-12

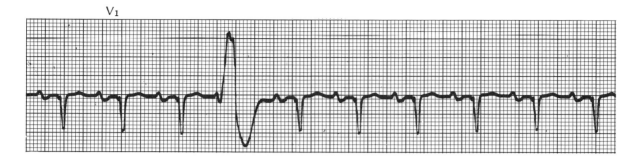

V_1

RATE: _____ (normal, bradycardia, or tachycardia). **RHYTHM:** _____ (regular or irregular) _____ (ventricular or supraventricular). **P-R INTERVAL:** _____ (too long, too short, or normal) _____ (absent P waves). **QRS DURATION:** _____ (normal or too long). **Q-T INTERVAL:** _____ (normal, too long, or too short). **P' WAVES:** _____ (present or absent). **JUNCTIONAL ECTOPIC BEATS:** _____ (present or absent). **VENTRICULAR ECTOPIC BEATS:** _____ (present or absent) _____ (unifocal or multifocal) _____ (frequent or infrequent) _____ (R on T). **Conclusion:** _____

ANALYSIS

RATE: 96/min. (normal). **RHYTHM:** irregular and supraventricular with ventricular. **P-R INTERVAL:** 0.22 sec. (too long). **QRS DURATION:** 0.09 sec. (normal). **Q-T INTERVAL:** 0.30 sec. (too short). **P' WAVES:** absent. **JUNCTIONAL ECTOPIC BEATS:** absent. **VENTRICULAR ECTOPIC BEATS:** present.

Conclusion: The type of PVC (end diastolic) seen in this tracing probably causes more diagnostic confusion than any other. This is mainly because it is preceded by a P wave (which does not conduct) and may sometimes be a fusion beat. The ventricles are partially captured by the sinus conducted beat and partially by the ventricular ectopic beat. If a PVC is more than 0.06 or 0.07 sec. premature, fusion is not possible since in that time the ventricular ectopic impulse would have completely depolarized the ventricles before the supraventricular impulse had time to enter.

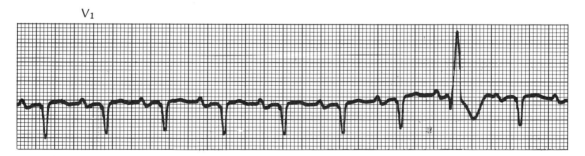

V_1

The tracing seen in the figure above is from the same patient. The same end diastolic PVC is present. However, this time it is a little later in the cycle and is now a fusion beat. If you had not noticed the change in P-R intervals, you might have mistaken this for intermittent bundle branch block (BBB).

End diastolic PVCs are not uncommon. It would be interesting to know what their relationship is to an elevation in left ventricular end diastolic pressure, as would occur in congestive heart failure. I know of no studies on this subject.

EXERCISE 4-13

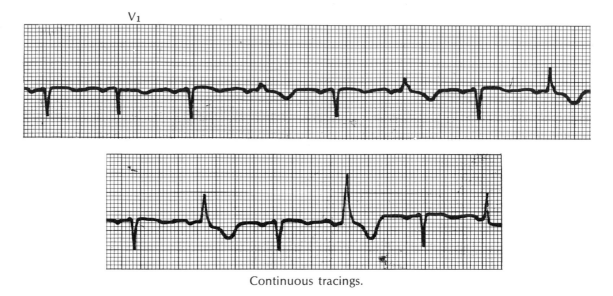

V₁

Continuous tracings.

RATE: _____ (normal, bradycardia, or tachycardia). **RHYTHM:** _____ (regular or irregular) _____ (ventricular or supraventricular). **P-R INTERVAL:** _____ (too long, too short, or normal) _____ (absent P waves). **QRS DURATION:** _____ (normal or too long). **Q-T INTERVAL:** _____ (normal, too long, or too short). **P' WAVES:** _____ (present or absent). **JUNCTIONAL ECTOPIC BEATS:** _____ (present or absent). **VENTRICULAR ECTOPIC BEATS:** _____ (present or absent) _____ (unifocal or multifocal) _____ (frequent or infrequent) _____ (R on T).
Conclusion: _____
_____

ANALYSIS

RATE: 78/min. (normal). **RHYTHM:** regular and supraventricular with ventricular. **P-R INTERVAL:** 0.15 sec. (normal). **QRS DURATION:** 0.09 sec. (normal). **Q-T INTERVAL:** 0.40 sec. (too long). **P' WAVES:** absent. **JUNCTIONAL ECTOPIC BEATS:** absent. **VENTRICULAR ECTOPIC BEATS:** present, unifocal, and frequent.

Conclusion: Here again are end diastolic PVCs. This time they occur in a bigeminal pattern, and almost all are fusion beats. Begin analyzing this arrhythmia by walking out the P waves. This is important because the sinus rhythm is perceived to be irregular when there are anomalous-looking beats following P waves. In this case it is absolutely regular. Go on to establish what is happening with A-V conduction. You will notice that the P-R shortens by 0.02 sec. with the broad beats. This is because a ventricular ectopic beat has fired before the sinus-conducted impulse reached the ventricles. Because the PVC is only slightly premature, it does not capture all of the ventricular myocardium. The sinus-conducted impulse will also partially conduct, causing a collision of opposing electrical currents, known as a fusion beat. Notice that all of the fusion beats are different from each other. This is because the ectopic focus and the sinus-conducted impulse never capture exactly the same amount of myocardium. Each beat is slightly different.

Notice the first fusion beat in the second complex, which is narrower than the flanking ones. Now skip across the tracing, looking at every other beat until finally in the second strip the tallest complex looks almost totally ectopic, although it is probably still a fusion beat.

The bigeminal end diastolic PVC presents one of the most confusing pictures in the arrhythmias. You should approach the tracing step by step in a logical manner until you have defined the function of the sinus node, A-V conduction, and ventricular conduction. You will meet with this arrhythmia again.

EXERCISE 4-14

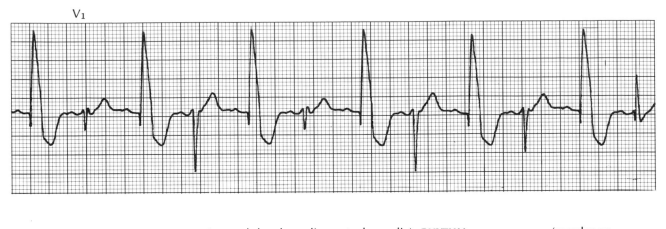

V₁

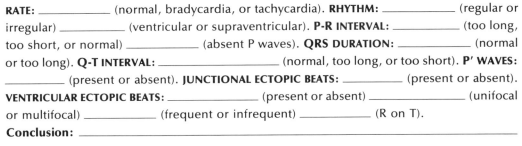

RATE: _____ (normal, bradycardia, or tachycardia). **RHYTHM:** _____ (regular or irregular) _____ (ventricular or supraventricular). **P-R INTERVAL:** _____ (too long, too short, or normal) _____ (absent P waves). **QRS DURATION:** _____ (normal or too long). **Q-T INTERVAL:** _____ (normal, too long, or too short). **P' WAVES:** _____ (present or absent). **JUNCTIONAL ECTOPIC BEATS:** _____ (present or absent).

VENTRICULAR ECTOPIC BEATS: _____ (present or absent) _____ (unifocal or multifocal) _____ (frequent or infrequent) _____ (R on T).

Conclusion: _____

ANALYSIS

RATE: 100/min. (normal). **RHYTHM:** regular and supraventricular with ventricular. **P-R INTERVAL:** 0.18 sec. (normal). **QRS DURATION:** 0.14 sec. (too long). **Q-T INTERVAL:** 0.36 sec. (too long). **P' WAVES:** absent. **JUNCTIONAL ECTOPIC BEATS:** absent. **VENTRICULAR ECTOPIC BEATS:** present, unifocal, and frequent.

Conclusion: Here again is a rhythm strip reflecting bigeminal end diastolic PVCs, which are fusion beats. At first you might think that the broad upright complexes are the ventricular ectopics. These are the sinus-conducted beats with an abnormally prolonged QRS. By walking out the P waves you will establish that the sinus rhythm is indeed regular even though it is perceived to be irregular. When you measure the P-R intervals, you will find that they are absolutely fixed before the broad upright beats but that they change before the narrower beats of varying morphology. These narrow beats are fusion beats caused by frequent ventricular ectopy and should be treated as such.

EXERCISE 4-15

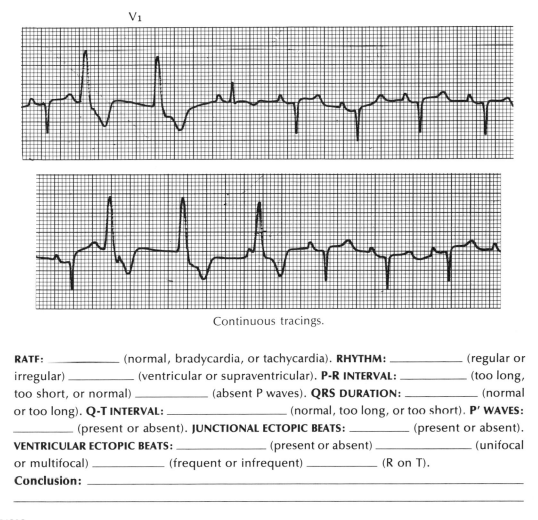

V₁

Continuous tracings.

RATE: _____ (normal, bradycardia, or tachycardia). RHYTHM: _____ (regular or irregular) _____ (ventricular or supraventricular). P-R INTERVAL: _____ (too long, too short, or normal) _____ (absent P waves). QRS DURATION: _____ (normal or too long). Q-T INTERVAL: _____ (normal, too long, or too short). P' WAVES: _____ (present or absent). JUNCTIONAL ECTOPIC BEATS: _____ (present or absent). VENTRICULAR ECTOPIC BEATS: _____ (present or absent) _____ (unifocal or multifocal) _____ (frequent or infrequent) _____ (R on T).

Conclusion: _____

_____

ANALYSIS

RATE: 75-88/min. (normal). RHYTHM: irregular and supraventricular with ventricular. P-R INTERVAL: 0.16 sec. (normal). QRS DURATION: 0.06 sec. (normal). Q-T INTERVAL: 0.34 sec. (normal). P' WAVES: absent. JUNCTIONAL ECTOPIC BEATS: absent. VENTRICULAR ECTOPIC BEATS: present, unifocal, and frequent.

Conclusion: Here is another kind of a PVC that can cause fusion beats. It is the accelerated idioventricular rhythm. This term implies that there is an area of enhanced automaticity within the ventricles that sometimes takes over as pacemaker at a rate of less than 100/min but at a rate that exceeds its own inherent one. This arrhythmia can manifest itself in different ways. Sometimes it appears to be more active and will begin with a very premature ventricular ectopic beat. At other times it will begin more passively in response to a pause in the sinus rhythm. However, it is not truly an escape mechanism, because its rate is too fast.

In the tracing above, there is an underlying sinus rate of 90/min. and an ectopic ventricular focus with an accelerated rate of 75/min. In the first tracing there are three PVCs from the accelerated ventricular focus; one of them is a fusion beat and follows a P wave (it is the fourth complex). In the second tracing (continuous from the first) three PVCs are again seen. The coupling interval for the first PVC of each group is the same. This may indicate that the arrhythmia is initiated by a reentry mechanism.

EXERCISE 4-16

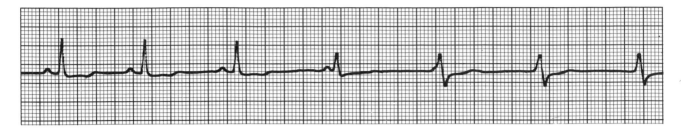

RATE: _____ (normal, bradycardia, or tachycardia). **RHYTHM:** _____ (regular or irregular) _____ (ventricular or supraventricular). **P-R INTERVAL:** _____ (too long, too short, or normal) _____ (absent P waves). **QRS DURATION:** _____ (normal or too long). **Q-T INTERVAL:** _____ (normal, too long, or too short). **P' WAVES:** _____ (present or absent). **JUNCTIONAL ECTOPIC BEATS:** _____ (present or absent). **VENTRICULAR ECTOPIC BEATS:** _____ (present or absent) _____ (unifocal or multifocal) _____ (frequent or infrequent) _____ (R on T).
Conclusion: _____

_____

ANALYSIS

RATE: 57-64/min. (bradycardia). RHYTHM: irregular and supraventricular with ventricular. P-R INTERVAL: 0.16 sec. (normal). QRS DURATION: 0.08 sec. (normal). Q-T INTERVAL: 0.40 sec. (normal). P' WAVES: absent. JUNCTIONAL ECTOPIC BEATS: absent. VENTRICULAR ECTOPIC BEATS: present, unifocal, and frequent.

Conclusion: This accelerated idioventricular rhythm begins with an end diastolic PVC, which is a fusion beat (fourth complex). There is an underlying sinus arrhythmia, and when the sinus rhythm slows down to 55/min., the accelerated ventricular focus manifests itself at a rate of 56/min. A junctional escape mechanism is ruled out because of the fusion beat and the broad ventricular complexes.

Whether or not to treat this arrhythmia is a controversial point among clinicians. It is an arrhythmia that often occurs with inferior wall myocardial infarction and has in years past been thought to be benign. Recently, however, some researchers have shown that it is not as benign as previously thought. Those physicians who agree with this concept will treat it aggressively. Those who do not will leave it untreated. The manner in which the arrhythmia is manifested is a consideration. For example, the tracing above shows a ventricular ectopic focus that took over only when the sinus node was slowing down. This is certainly more passive and less threatening than the accelerated idioventricular rhythm shown in exercise 4-15.

EXERCISE 4-17

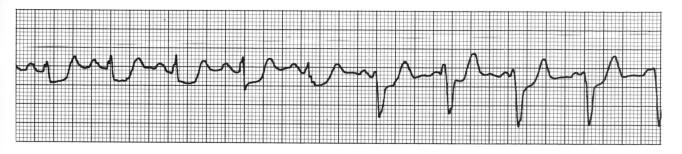

RATE: _____ (normal, bradycardia, or tachycardia). **RHYTHM:** _____ (regular or irregular) _____ (ventricular or supraventricular). **P-R INTERVAL:** _____ (too long, too short, or normal) _____ (absent P waves). **QRS DURATION:** _____ (normal or too long). **Q-T INTERVAL:** _____ (normal, too long, or too short). **P' WAVES:** _____ (present or absent). **JUNCTIONAL ECTOPIC BEATS:** _____ (present or absent). **VENTRICULAR ECTOPIC BEATS:** _____ (present or absent) _____ (unifocal or multifocal) _____ (frequent or infrequent) _____ (R on T).
Conclusion: _____
_____

ANALYSIS

RATE: 80-88/min. (normal). **RHYTHM:** regular and supraventricular/ventricular. **P-R INTERVAL:** 0.18 sec. (normal). **QRS DURATION:** 0.08 sec. (normal). **Q-T INTERVAL:** 0.38 sec. (normal). **P' WAVES:** absent. **JUNCTIONAL ECTOPIC BEATS:** absent. **VENTRICULAR ECTOPIC BEATS:** present, unifocal, and frequent.

Conclusion: Here again, an accelerated idioventricular focus takes over as an end diastolic PVC, which is a fusion beat (fourth complex). There are probably four more fusion beats before there is full capture of the ventricles by the ectopic focus.

EXERCISE 4-18

II

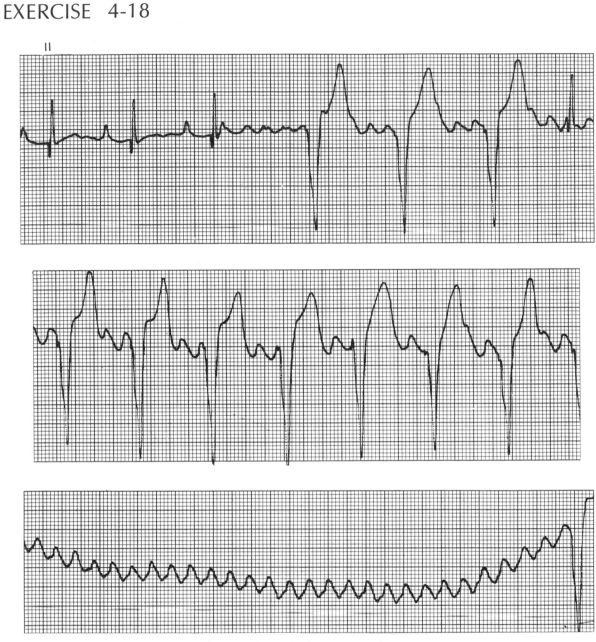

Same patient. Tracings not continuous.

RATE: _____ (normal, bradycardia, or tachycardia). **RHYTHM:** _____ (regular or irregular) _____ (ventricular or supraventricular). **P-R INTERVAL:** _____ (too long, too short, or normal) _____ (absent P waves). **QRS DURATION:** _____ (normal or too long). **Q-T INTERVAL:** _____ (normal, too long, or too short). **P' WAVES:** _____ (present or absent). **JUNCTIONAL ECTOPIC BEATS:** _____ (present or absent). **VENTRICULAR ECTOPIC BEATS:** _____ (present or absent) _____ (unifocal or multifocal) _____ (frequent or infrequent) _____ (R on T).
Conclusion: _____

_____

ANALYSIS

RATE: 70-75/min. (normal). RHYTHM: irregular, supraventricular, and ventricular. P-R INTERVAL: 0.28 sec. (too long). QRS DURATION: 0.10 sec. (normal). Q-T INTERVAL: 0.40 sec. (normal). P' WAVES: present and premature. JUNCTIONAL ECTOPIC BEATS: absent. VENTRICULAR ECTOPIC BEATS: present and escape.

Conclusion: The accelerated idioventricular rhythm in this tracing occurs against a background of atrial flutter. The onset of the first tracing shows a first-degree A-V block with normal intraventricular conduction and a prominent U wave, perhaps reflective of hypokalemia. A PAC occurs just after the third ventricular complex and triggers atrial flutter at a rate of 300/min. Killip's rule states that if a premature atrial complex ends a cycle by less than 50%, it is likely to cause a more serious atrial ectopic rhythm. If the P-P' interval is more than 60% of the P-P interval, there will be no serious consequences. This rule is certainly well illustrated in this tracing. The P-P' interval is less than 50% of the P-P interval, and atrial flutter ensues. The first ventricular complex to occur after the onset of atrial flutter represents an accelerated idioventricular rhythm. One complex can be seen to have been conducted from the atrial pacemaker (capture), but the main ventricular rhythm is dissociated from the atrial rhythm. Even if the onset of the atrial flutter had not been available to you, this diagnosis would still have been evident because of the changing relationship of the flutter wave to the R wave and because of the absolute regularity of the ventricular rhythm. In the second tracing, the flutter waves are not easily seen because of a further acceleration of the ventricular pacemaker. This tracing should impress you with the importance of determining whether the P waves belong to the QRS or not and whether the T waves are all of the same shape. Remember that a P' wave will usually distort a T wave if it occurs at the same time.

The third tracing is from the same patient and is presented here to show you clearly the ECG of atrial flutter. Notice that there is no pause in the sawtooth pattern and that the P' waves (the negative component) are absolutely regular. This should be recalled when you are determining the conduction ratio in atrial flutter. The P' waves should be walked out so that the flutter waves hidden by the QRS-T complex will not be missed.

EXERCISE 4-19

V_1

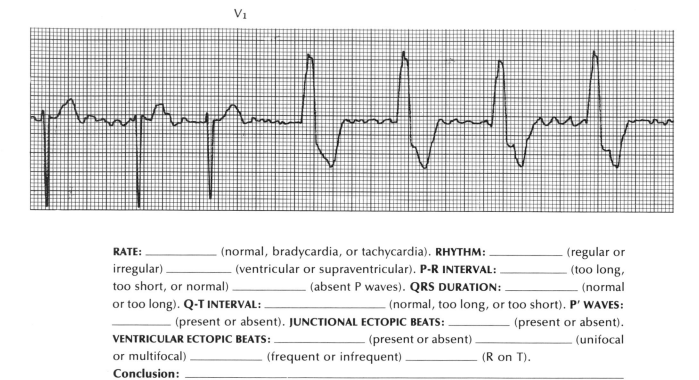

RATE: _____ (normal, bradycardia, or tachycardia). **RHYTHM:** _____ (regular or irregular) _____ (ventricular or supraventricular). **P-R INTERVAL:** _____ (too long, too short, or normal) _____ (absent P waves). **QRS DURATION:** _____ (normal or too long). **Q-T INTERVAL:** _____ (normal, too long, or too short). **P' WAVES:** _____ (present or absent). **JUNCTIONAL ECTOPIC BEATS:** _____ (present or absent). **VENTRICULAR ECTOPIC BEATS:** _____ (present or absent) _____ (unifocal or multifocal) _____ (frequent or infrequent) _____ (R on T). **Conclusion:** _____

ANALYSIS

RATE: 60-65/min. (normal). RHYTHM: irregular supraventricular and regular ventricular. P-R INTERVAL: absent P waves. QRS DURATION: 0.08 sec. (normal). Q-T INTERVAL: varies (normal). P' WAVES: absent. JUNCTIONAL ECTOPIC BEATS: absent. VENTRICULAR ECTOPIC BEATS: present, unifocal, and frequent.

Conclusion: The underlying rhythm here is atrial fibrillation. There is an accelerated idioventricular focus in the left ventricle that takes over at a rate of 60/min.

At the beginning of the tracing there is an appropriately irregular ventricular response. In atrial fibrillation, absolutely regular and/or very broad ventricular complexes are inappropriate and indicate an idioventricular mechanism. It is "accelerated" because the inherent rate of pacemakers below the branching portion of the bundle of His is less than 40/min.

EXERCISE 4-20

V₁

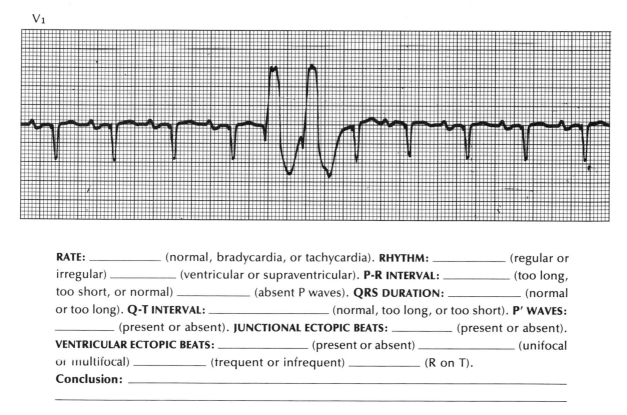

RATE: _____ (normal, bradycardia, or tachycardia). **RHYTHM:** _____ (regular or irregular) _____ (ventricular or supraventricular). **P-R INTERVAL:** _____ (too long, too short, or normal) _____ (absent P waves). **QRS DURATION:** _____ (normal or too long). **Q-T INTERVAL:** _____ (normal, too long, or too short). **P′ WAVES:** _____ (present or absent). **JUNCTIONAL ECTOPIC BEATS:** _____ (present or absent). **VENTRICULAR ECTOPIC BEATS:** _____ (present or absent) _____ (unifocal or multifocal) _____ (frequent or infrequent) _____ (R on T).
Conclusion: _____

_____

ANALYSIS

RATE: 94-110/min. (tachycardia). **RHYTHM:** irregular and supraventricular with ventricular. **P-R INTERVAL:** 0.22 sec. (too long). **QRS DURATION:** 0.08 sec. (normal). **Q-T INTERVAL:** 0.28 sec. (too short). **P′ WAVES:** absent. **JUNCTIONAL ECTOPIC BEATS:** absent. **VENTRICULAR ECTOPIC BEATS:** present, unifocal, and paired.

Conclusion: The back to back, left ventricular PVCs in this tracing are a cause for concern and should be treated aggressively. When one PVC follows another in rapid succession, the second of the two is necessarily very close to the T wave of the preceding beat. This means that it will capture the ventricles when the membrane potential has not yet reached its optimal level for normal uniform conduction. Ventricular fibrillation may be the result of such a sequence. The second PVC has retrograde conduction to the atria. The normal complex following it is a reciprocal beat.

This patient also has a first-degree heart block, detected by measuring the P-R interval, which should not exceed 0.20 sec. Heart block is discussed and illustrated in Chapter 5.

EXERCISE 4-21

V₁

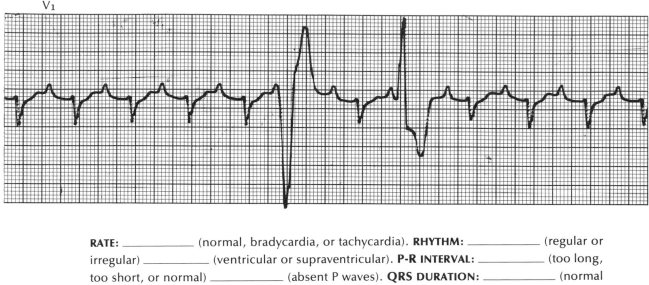

RATE: _____ (normal, bradycardia, or tachycardia). **RHYTHM:** _____ (regular or irregular) _____ (ventricular or supraventricular). **P-R INTERVAL:** _____ (too long, too short, or normal) _____ (absent P waves). **QRS DURATION:** _____ (normal or too long). **Q-T INTERVAL:** _____ (normal, too long, or too short). **P' WAVES:** _____ (present or absent). **JUNCTIONAL ECTOPIC BEATS:** _____ (present or absent).

VENTRICULAR ECTOPIC BEATS: _____ (present or absent) _____ (unifocal or multifocal) _____ (frequent or infrequent) _____ (R on T).

Conclusion: _____

ANALYSIS

RATE: 98-100/min. (normal). **RHYTHM:** irregular and supraventricular with ventricular. **P-R INTERVAL:** 0.28 sec. (too long). **QRS DURATION:** 0.08 sec. (normal). **Q-T INTERVAL:** difficult to determine. **P' WAVES:** absent. **JUNCTIONAL ECTOPIC BEATS:** absent. **VENTRICULAR ECTOPIC BEATS:** present, multifocal, and frequent.

Conclusion: The two PVCs in this tracing are decidedly from different foci. Multifocal PVCs are more threatening than unifocal and should be treated aggressively. The first PVC is right ventricular in origin, and the second is left ventricular. Both of them occur toward the end of diastole. Because this patient also has first-degree heart block with a P-R interval of 0.28 sec., there is no chance of the second PVC being a fusion beat. In order for fusion to occur, the ventricular ectopic beat cannot be more than 0.06 or 0.07 sec. premature. The second PVC is 0.16 sec. premature and completely captures the ventricles before the sinus P wave can conduct across the A-V node.

EXERCISE 4-22

V₁

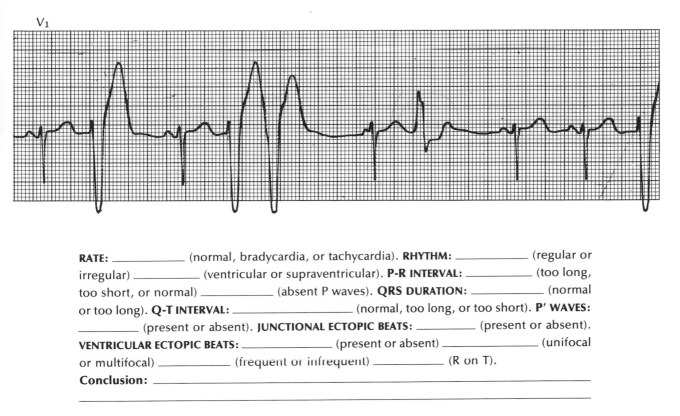

RATE: _____ (normal, bradycardia, or tachycardia). **RHYTHM:** _____ (regular or irregular) _____ (ventricular or supraventricular). **P-R INTERVAL:** _____ (too long, too short, or normal) _____ (absent P waves). **QRS DURATION:** _____ (normal or too long). **Q-T INTERVAL:** _____ (normal, too long, or too short). **P' WAVES:** _____ (present or absent). **JUNCTIONAL ECTOPIC BEATS:** _____ (present or absent).

VENTRICULAR ECTOPIC BEATS: _____ (present or absent) _____ (unifocal or multifocal) _____ (frequent or infrequent) _____ (R on T).

Conclusion: _____

_____

ANALYSIS

RATE: 90/min. (normal). **RHYTHM:** irregular and supraventricular/ventricular. **P-R INTERVAL:** 0.12 sec. (normal). **QRS DURATION:** 0.09 sec. (normal). **Q-T INTERVAL:** 0.36 sec. (normal). **P' WAVES:** absent. **JUNCTIONAL ECTOPIC BEATS:** present and escape. **VENTRICULAR ECTOPIC BEATS:** present, multifocal, frequent, and paired.

Conclusion: The ventricular ectopy manifested in this tracing is primarily right ventricular; however, because they occur in pairs, are so frequent, and are multifocal (left ventricular as well), treatment will be aggressive.

There is a junctional escape beat following the back to back PVCs.

EXERCISE 4-23

V₁

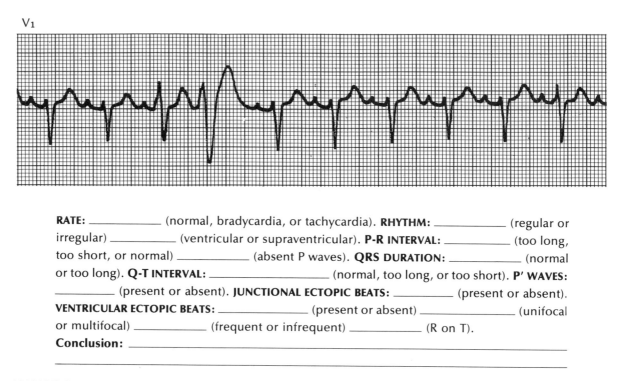

RATE: _____ (normal, bradycardia, or tachycardia). **RHYTHM:** _____ (regular or irregular) _____ (ventricular or supraventricular). **P-R INTERVAL:** _____ (too long, too short, or normal) _____ (absent P waves). **QRS DURATION:** _____ (normal or too long). **Q-T INTERVAL:** _____ (normal, too long, or too short). **P' WAVES:** _____ (present or absent). **JUNCTIONAL ECTOPIC BEATS:** _____ (present or absent). **VENTRICULAR ECTOPIC BEATS:** _____ (present or absent) _____ (unifocal or multifocal) _____ (frequent or infrequent) _____ (R on T).
Conclusion: _____
_____

ANALYSIS

RATE: 100-105/min. (tachycardia). **RHYTHM:** irregular and supraventricular with ventricular. **P-R INTERVAL:** 0.18 sec. (normal). **QRS DURATION:** 0.10 sec. (normal). **Q-T INTERVAL:** 0.36 sec. (too long). **P' WAVES:** absent. **JUNCTIONAL ECTOPIC BEATS:** absent. **VENTRICULAR ECTOPIC BEATS:** present, unifocal, and paired.

Conclusion: There are two PVCs in this tracing. They are back to back, and the first of the pair is an end diastolic fusion beat (third complex). A borderline sinus tachycardia is also present.

EXERCISE 4-24

II

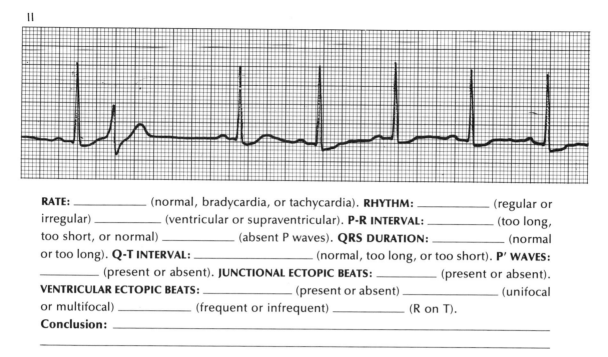

RATE: _____ (normal, bradycardia, or tachycardia). **RHYTHM:** _____ (regular or irregular) _____ (ventricular or supraventricular). **P-R INTERVAL:** _____ (too long, too short, or normal) _____ (absent P waves). **QRS DURATION:** _____ (normal or too long). **Q-T INTERVAL:** _____ (normal, too long, or too short). **P' WAVES:** _____ (present or absent). **JUNCTIONAL ECTOPIC BEATS:** _____ (present or absent). **VENTRICULAR ECTOPIC BEATS:** _____ (present or absent) _____ (unifocal or multifocal) _____ (frequent or infrequent) _____ (R on T).
Conclusion: _____

ANALYSIS

RATE: 70-75/min. (normal). RHYTHM: irregular and supraventricular with ventricular. P-R INTERVAL: 0.20 sec. (normal). QRS DURATION: 0.08 sec. (normal). Q-T INTERVAL: 0.35 sec. (normal). P' WAVES: absent. JUNCTIONAL ECTOPIC BEATS: absent. VENTRICULAR ECTOPIC BEATS: present, with R-on-T phenomenon.

Conclusion: When the ventricular complex occurs during the T wave, as in this tracing, it is referred to as the "R-on-T phenomenon." This patient should be treated aggressively with antiarrhythmics and watched closely, with the possibility kept in mind that the next PVC occurring during the refractory period of the ventricles may trigger ventricular fibrillation.

During the T wave the ventricular cells are repolarizing. In some cells the membrane potential is high enough to accept a stimulus but will do so sluggishly. This will in turn reflect in conduction velocity, which will be slow. Other cells will not have repolarized enough to accept a stimulus at all, and current flow will be blocked in this part of the heart. The result, then, of a stimulus occurring during the T wave, and especially at the peak of the T wave, may be ventricular tachycardia or fibrillation.

EXERCISE 4-25

II

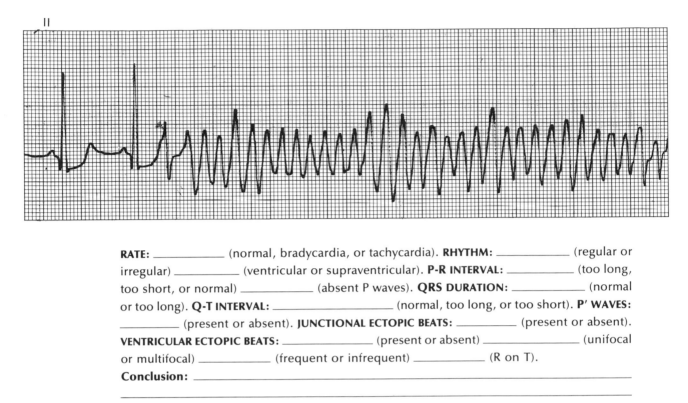

RATE: _____ (normal, bradycardia, or tachycardia). **RHYTHM:** _____ (regular or irregular) _____ (ventricular or supraventricular). **P-R INTERVAL:** _____ (too long, too short, or normal) _____ (absent P waves). **QRS DURATION:** _____ (normal or too long). **Q-T INTERVAL:** _____ (normal, too long, or too short). **P' WAVES:** _____ (present or absent). **JUNCTIONAL ECTOPIC BEATS:** _____ (present or absent).

VENTRICULAR ECTOPIC BEATS: _____ (present or absent) _____ (unifocal or multifocal) _____ (frequent or infrequent) _____ (R on T).

Conclusion: _____

ANALYSIS

RATE: 75/min. (first two beats). RHYTHM: irregular and ventricular. P-R INTERVAL: 0.12 sec. (normal). QRS DURATION: 0.09 sec. (normal). Q-T INTERVAL: 0.40 sec. (too long). P' WAVES: absent. JUNCTIONAL ECTOPIC BEATS: absent. VENTRICULAR ECTOPIC BEATS: present, with R-on-T phenomenon.

Conclusion: This patient exhibits the R-on-T phenomenon, which sparks ventricular flutter and fibrillation. There is an excessively long Q-T interval, indicating a lengthening of the refractory period. If the increment is in phase 3 of the action potential, the patient is more vulnerable for a longer period.

The rhythm following the first PVC has some order to it and may be called a ventricular flutter. However, it will quickly deteriorate into fibrillation. In this case the distinction is purely academic since the patient is clinically dead with either arrhythmia.

As soon as ventricular tachycardia or fibrillation begins, the electrolyte balance of the patient quickly deteriorates to acidosis.

EXERCISE 4-26

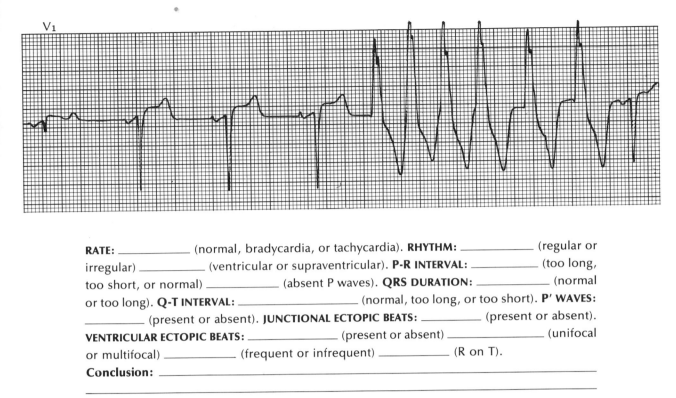

V₁

RATE: _____ (normal, bradycardia, or tachycardia). **RHYTHM:** _____ (regular or irregular) _____ (ventricular or supraventricular). **P-R INTERVAL:** _____ (too long, too short, or normal) _____ (absent P waves). **QRS DURATION:** _____ (normal or too long). **Q-T INTERVAL:** _____ (normal, too long, or too short). **P′ WAVES:** _____ (present or absent). **JUNCTIONAL ECTOPIC BEATS:** _____ (present or absent). **VENTRICULAR ECTOPIC BEATS:** _____ (present or absent) _____ (unifocal or multifocal) _____ (frequent or infrequent) _____ (R on T).

Conclusion: _____

_____

ANALYSIS

RATE: 63-154/min. (tachycardia). **RHYTHM:** irregular and supraventricular/ventricular. **P-R INTERVAL:** 0.13 sec. (normal). **QRS DURATION:** 0.10 sec. (normal). **Q-T INTERVAL:** 0.40 sec. (normal). **P′ WAVES:** present. **JUNCTIONAL ECTOPIC BEATS:** absent. **VENTRICULAR ECTOPIC BEATS:** present, unifocal, and frequent.

Conclusion: This is a paroxysmal left ventricular tachycardia. The very first complex is a fusion beat. Notice how narrow it is and how decreased the amplitude is compared with the three sinus-conducted beats that follow. A burst of ventricular tachycardia follows. There is a P wave seen immediately after the last ventricular ectopic beat. It probably represents retrograde conduction from the ventricles. It is followed by normal ventricular conduction, in this case a reciprocal beat.

EXERCISE 4-27

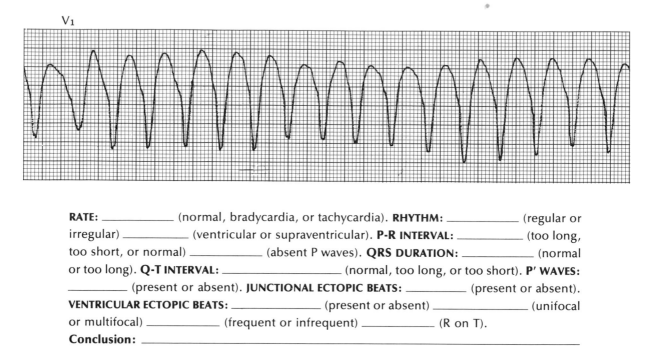

V₁

RATE: _____ (normal, bradycardia, or tachycardia). **RHYTHM:** _____ (regular or irregular) _____ (ventricular or supraventricular). **P-R INTERVAL:** _____ (too long, too short, or normal) _____ (absent P waves). **QRS DURATION:** _____ (normal or too long). **Q-T INTERVAL:** _____ (normal, too long, or too short). **P' WAVES:** _____ (present or absent). **JUNCTIONAL ECTOPIC BEATS:** _____ (present or absent). **VENTRICULAR ECTOPIC BEATS:** _____ (present or absent) _____ (unifocal or multifocal) _____ (frequent or infrequent) _____ (R on T).
Conclusion: _____
_____

ANALYSIS

RATE: 170/min. (tachycardia). **RHYTHM:** regular and ventricular. **P-R INTERVAL:** not applicable. **QRS DURATION:** 0.16 sec. (too long). **Q-T INTERVAL:** approximately 0.36 sec. **P' WAVES:** absent. **JUNCTIONAL ECTOPIC BEATS:** absent. **VENTRICULAR ECTOPIC BEATS:** present, unifocal, and frequent.

Conclusion: This is ventricular tachycardia, an extreme emergency. A tachycardia will severely compromise the already ischemic myocardium, depreciate general hemodynamics, and precipitate ventricular fibrillation. The mechanism involved is either a single focus with enhanced automaticity, or it is a reentry mechanism. In the latter case the episode would have been sparked by a single PVC, occurring at just the right time in the cardiac cycle.

EXERCISE 4-28

V₁

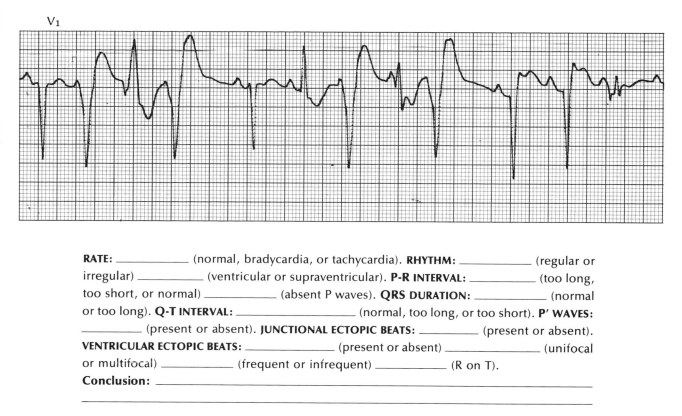

RATE: _____ (normal, bradycardia, or tachycardia). **RHYTHM:** _____ (regular or irregular) _____ (ventricular or supraventricular). **P-R INTERVAL:** _____ (too long, too short, or normal) _____ (absent P waves). **QRS DURATION:** _____ (normal or too long). **Q-T INTERVAL:** _____ (normal, too long, or too short). **P′ WAVES:** _____ (present or absent). **JUNCTIONAL ECTOPIC BEATS:** _____ (present or absent). **VENTRICULAR ECTOPIC BEATS:** _____ (present or absent) _____ (unifocal or multifocal) _____ (frequent or infrequent) _____ (R on T).
Conclusion: _____
_____

ANALYSIS

RATE: 110/min. (tachycardia). **RHYTHM:** irregular and primarily ventricular. **P-R INTERVAL:** 0.16 sec. (normal). **QRS DURATION:** 0.08 sec. (normal). **Q-T INTERVAL:** varies (normal). **P′ WAVES:** absent. **JUNCTIONAL ECTOPIC BEATS:** absent. **VENTRICULAR ECTOPIC BEATS:** present, multifocal, and frequent.

Conclusion: There are frequent multifocal PVCs in this tracing. Sometimes they are end diastolic fusion beats, and therefore it is difficult to pick out the sinus-conducted beats. There is a sinus-conducted beat at the very beginning of the tracing. The fifth beat from the beginning is also a sinus-conducted beat. Evidence of the dual focus is seen right after the first normal beat. There is a right and then a left ventricular PVC. Another right ventricular PVC follows, and it almost looks as though you will see an established bidirectional ventricular tachycardia, which is commonly caused by digitalis toxicity.

Some authorities do not use the term "multifocal" but prefer "multiform" instead.[68] They feel that ventricular ectopics exhibiting more than one morphology in the same heart may actually be one focus with different wave fronts.

EXERCISE 4-29

V₁

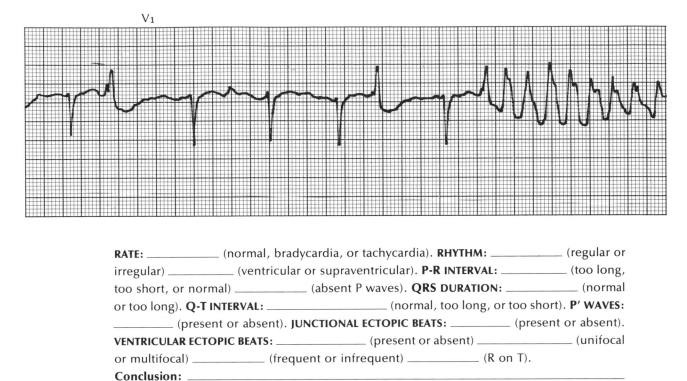

RATE: _____ (normal, bradycardia, or tachycardia). **RHYTHM:** _____ (regular or irregular) _____ (ventricular or supraventricular). **P-R INTERVAL:** _____ (too long, too short, or normal) _____ (absent P waves). **QRS DURATION:** _____ (normal or too long). **Q-T INTERVAL:** _____ (normal, too long, or too short). **P' WAVES:** _____ (present or absent). **JUNCTIONAL ECTOPIC BEATS:** _____ (present or absent). **VENTRICULAR ECTOPIC BEATS:** _____ (present or absent) _____ (unifocal or multifocal) _____ (frequent or infrequent) _____ (R on T). **Conclusion:** _____

_____

ANALYSIS

RATE: 80-160/min. (tachycardia). RHYTHM: irregular and supraventricular/ventricular. P-R INTERVAL: absent P waves. QRS DURATION: 0.09 sec. (normal). Q-T INTERVAL: difficult to determine. P' WAVES: absent. JUNCTIONAL ECTOPIC BEATS: absent. VENTRICULAR ECTOPIC BEATS: present, unifocal, and frequent.

Conclusion: In this tracing there is an underlying atrial fibrillation with frequent left ventricular PVCs, which deteriorate into ventricular tachycardia. This patient would have already lost 20% of his cardiac output with the atrial fibrillation. The ventricular tachycardia will further seriously compromise hemodynamics and should be converted immediately.

EXERCISE 4-30

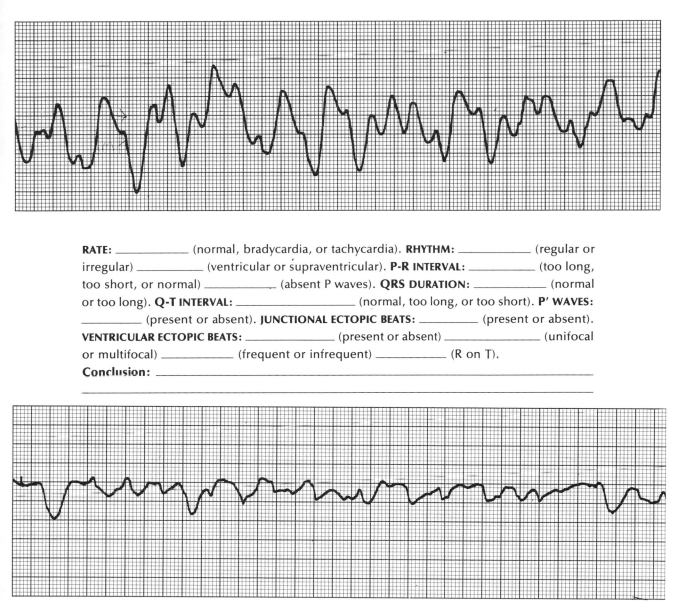

RATE: _____ (normal, bradycardia, or tachycardia). **RHYTHM:** _____ (regular or irregular) _____ (ventricular or supraventricular). **P-R INTERVAL:** _____ (too long, too short, or normal) _____ (absent P waves). **QRS DURATION:** _____ (normal or too long). **Q-T INTERVAL:** _____ (normal, too long, or too short). **P' WAVES:** _____ (present or absent). **JUNCTIONAL ECTOPIC BEATS:** _____ (present or absent). **VENTRICULAR ECTOPIC BEATS:** _____ (present or absent) _____ (unifocal or multifocal) _____ (frequent or infrequent) _____ (R on T).
Conclusion: _____
_____

ANALYSIS

This totally disorganized electrical pattern represents ventricular fibrillation. The patient should be defibrillated immediately. In this arrhythmia the clinical picture is such that the tracing is seldom misinterpreted. The figure above offers you another ventricular fibrillation to study. Note the total lack of any wave form that is repeated in a regular fashion. The ventricles are quivering (fibrillating). There is depolarization and repolarization but not in an organized fashion. Single cells and small groups of cells work independently of each other. The ventricles, of course, do not pump blood.

EXERCISE 4-31

II

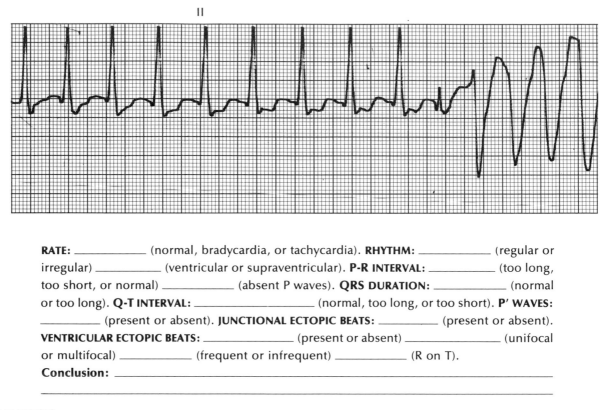

RATE: _____ (normal, bradycardia, or tachycardia). **RHYTHM:** _____ (regular or irregular) _____ (ventricular or supraventricular). **P-R INTERVAL:** _____ (too long, too short, or normal) _____ (absent P waves). **QRS DURATION:** _____ (normal or too long). **Q-T INTERVAL:** _____ (normal, too long, or too short). **P' WAVES:** _____ (present or absent). **JUNCTIONAL ECTOPIC BEATS:** _____ (present or absent). **VENTRICULAR ECTOPIC BEATS:** _____ (present or absent) _____ (unifocal or multifocal) _____ (frequent or infrequent) _____ (R on T). **Conclusion:** _____
_____

ANALYSIS

RATE: 115-150/min. (tachycardia). **RHYTHM:** irregular and primarily ventricular. **P-R INTERVAL:** absent P waves. **QRS DURATION:** 0.16 sec. (too long). **Q-T INTERVAL:** 0.44 sec. (too long). **P' WAVES:** absent. **JUNCTIONAL ECTOPIC BEATS:** present and premature. **VENTRICULAR ECTOPIC BEATS:** present, unifocal, and frequent.

Conclusion: This ventricular tachycardia begins with a ventricular fusion beat (the tenth complex). The beginning of the tracing reveals no P waves (atrial fibrillation). The first two or three ventricular complexes are appropriately irregular, after which they become regular. This may be a manifestation of digitalis toxicity. In atrial fibrillation digitalis excess may manifest as complete heart block and nonparoxysmal junctional tachycardia, as is seen in this patient.

EXERCISE 4-32

V₁

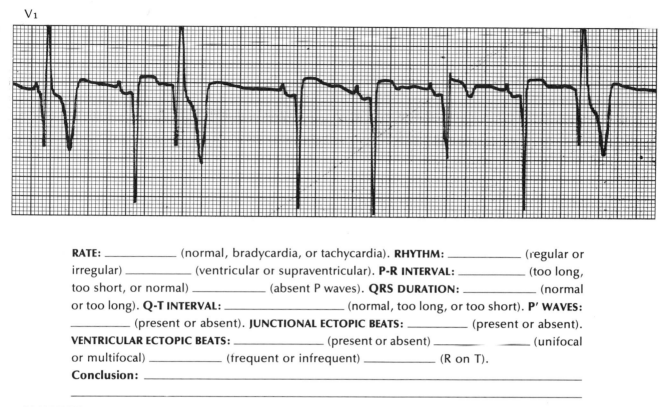

RATE: _____ (normal, bradycardia, or tachycardia). **RHYTHM:** _____ (regular or irregular) _____ (ventricular or supraventricular). **P-R INTERVAL:** _____ (too long, too short, or normal) _____ (absent P waves). **QRS DURATION:** _____ (normal or too long). **Q-T INTERVAL:** _____ (normal, too long, or too short). **P' WAVES:** _____ (present or absent). **JUNCTIONAL ECTOPIC BEATS:** _____ (present or absent). **VENTRICULAR ECTOPIC BEATS:** _____ (present or absent) _____ (unifocal or multifocal) _____ (frequent or infrequent) _____ (R on T). **Conclusion:** _____

_____

ANALYSIS

RATE: 70-75/min. (normal). **RHYTHM:** irregular and supraventricular with ventricular. **P-R INTERVAL:** 0.16 sec. (normal). **QRS DURATION:** 0.08 sec. (normal). **Q-T INTERVAL** 0.29 sec. (too short). **P' WAVES:** absent. **JUNCTIONAL ECTOPIC BEATS:** absent. **VENTRICULAR ECTOPIC BEATS:** present, unifocal, and frequent.

Conclusion: There is a ventricular parasystolic focus in this heart. Parasystole is manifested with ventricular ectopics that have no fixed coupling. Fusion beats will also be seen. This is an example of the classic parasystole, especially since the ectopic rhythm can be exactly walked out (the ectopic R-R intervals are exact multiples). This last criterion, however, is not necessary for parasystole to be present.[69]

A parasystolic focus is so named because it is a dual rhythm, the ectopic focus being protected from depolarization from outside stimulus, such as the sinus-conducted impulse. If the parasystolic focus were not protected, it would reset itself each time the normal ventricular impulse depolarized it. Its rate would then be irregular. This protection is accomplished by an area of decremental conduction and one-way conduction surrounding the area of enhanced automaticity. This means that the ectopic impulse can exit into the normal myocardium but that the normal ventricular impulse cannot penetrate the ischemic area.

In the above tracing the first beat is an end diastolic PVC, followed by a normal beat and then another PVC, both with different coupling intervals. If you use the ectopic R-R interval as a measure, you will find that the next expected beat (supposing a protected focus) would have occurred in the T wave of the fourth beat. Then, right on time, the next PVC is a fusion beat. The tracing ends with another PVC, also right on time. When the PVCs are exactly coupled to a preceding beat, you can at least predict where the ectopic beat will fall each time. With the parasystolic focus the PVC can easily fall on a T wave.

EXERCISE 4-33

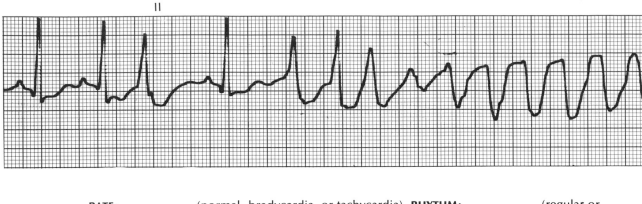

II

RATE: _____ (normal, bradycardia, or tachycardia). **RHYTHM:** _____ (regular or irregular) _____ (ventricular or supraventricular). **P-R INTERVAL:** _____ (too long, too short, or normal) _____ (absent P waves). **QRS DURATION:** _____ (normal or too long). **Q-T INTERVAL:** _____ (normal, too long, or too short). **P' WAVES:** _____ (present or absent). **JUNCTIONAL ECTOPIC BEATS:** _____ (present or absent). **VENTRICULAR ECTOPIC BEATS:** _____ (present or absent) _____ (unifocal or multifocal) _____ (frequent or infrequent) _____ (R on T).
Conclusion: _____

ANALYSIS

RATE: 90-150/min. (tachycardia). **RHYTHM:** irregular and supraventricular/ventricular. **P-R INTERVAL:** 0.15 sec. (normal). **QRS DURATION:** 0.14 sec. (too long). **Q-T INTERVAL:** 0.47 sec. (too long). **P' WAVES:** absent. **JUNCTIONAL ECTOPIC BEATS:** absent. **VENTRICULAR ECTOPIC BEATS:** present, unifocal, and frequent.

Conclusion: Here is a parasystolic focus in which the PVCs are firing on the T wave. The third complex is on a T wave. This is further complicated by an excessively long Q-T interval (refractory period). The parasystolic focus manifests itself again after the fourth beat, and ventricular tachycardia ensues.

EXERCISE 4-34

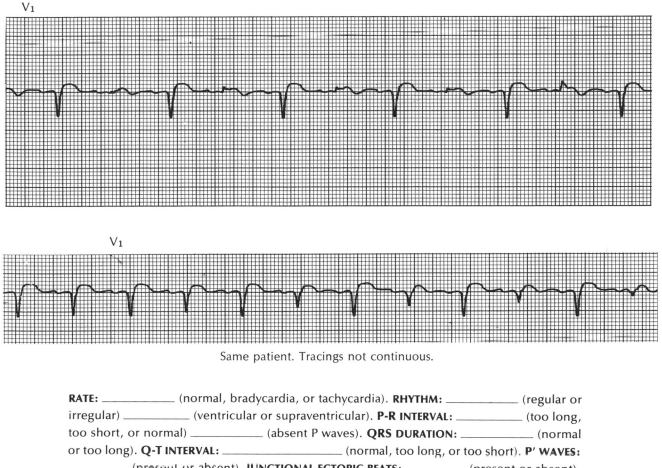

V₁

V₁

Same patient. Tracings not continuous.

RATE: _____ (normal, bradycardia, or tachycardia). **RHYTHM:** _____ (regular or irregular) _____ (ventricular or supraventricular). **P-R INTERVAL:** _____ (too long, too short, or normal) _____ (absent P waves). **QRS DURATION:** _____ (normal or too long). **Q-T INTERVAL:** _____ (normal, too long, or too short). **P′ WAVES:** _____ (present or absent). **JUNCTIONAL ECTOPIC BEATS:** _____ (present or absent). **VENTRICULAR ECTOPIC BEATS:** _____ (present or absent) _____ (unifocal or multifocal) _____ (frequent or infrequent) _____ (R on T).
Conclusion: _____
_____

ANALYSIS

RATE: 100/min. (normal). **RHYTHM:** regular and supraventricular/ventricular. **P-R INTERVAL:** 0.16 sec. (normal). **QRS DURATION:** 0.08 sec. (normal). **Q-T INTERVAL:** 0.24 sec. (too short). **P′ WAVES:** absent. **JUNCTIONAL ECTOPIC BEATS:** absent. **VENTRICULAR ECTOPIC BEATS:** present, unifocal, and frequent.

Conclusion: This patient has bigeminal, end diastolic PVCs. All of them are fusion beats and they do not look like PVCs at all. Somebody might even mistake this for electrical alternans. You can see the varying degrees of ventricular fusion every other beat, especially in the second tracing from the same patient. The second beat in the tracing is a fusion, but it is not as apparent as the fourth beat. After this, every other complex has varying degrees of fusion until the complex is almost isoelectric. The only thing that can cause ventricular fusion in a sinus-conducted beat is a ventricular ectopic focus.

CHAPTER 5

ATRIOVENTRICULAR HEART BLOCK AND PACEMAKERS

This chapter deals again with the A-V junction. In Chapter 3 you became proficient in recognizing ectopic junctional beats and rhythms, both escape and premature. Now we will review A-V heart block. In the exercises that follow, you are given practice in recognizing first-degree, second-degree, and third-degree A-V heart block, pacemaker rhythms, and pacemaker malfunction.

In first-degree heart block all impulses are conducted, but with a prolonged A-V conduction time (P-R interval). From the beginning of this book you have been measuring the P-R interval and determining whether or not it is too long. If it is beyond 0.20 sec. and if all beats are conducted, first-degree heart block is present.

In second-degree heart block some P waves are not conducted. There are two types of second-degree block. In type I (Wenckebach) the P-R intervals increase until a P wave is not conducted. Then the cycle begins again. In type II all the P-R intervals are the same. The Wenckebach phenomenon is usually a function of the A-V node and rarely a function of the atrial or His-Purkinje system.[76,79] Type II block is most frequently an infra-His phenomenon, involving the bundle braches.[76,77]

In third-degree heart block there is no conduction at all between the atria and the ventricles. This block is pathological and not functional, as it would be in A-V dissociation. Briefly, if conduction is possible and does not take place, third-degree heart block is present.

EXERCISE 5-1

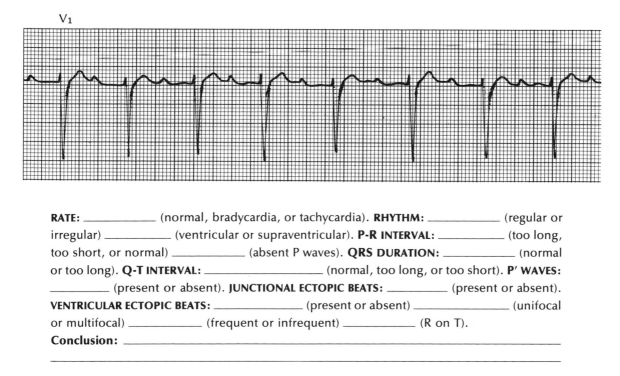

V₁

RATE: _____ (normal, bradycardia, or tachycardia). **RHYTHM:** _____ (regular or irregular) _____ (ventricular or supraventricular). **P-R INTERVAL:** _____ (too long, too short, or normal) _____ (absent P waves). **QRS DURATION:** _____ (normal or too long). **Q-T INTERVAL:** _____ (normal, too long, or too short). **P' WAVES:** _____ (present or absent). **JUNCTIONAL ECTOPIC BEATS:** _____ (present or absent). **VENTRICULAR ECTOPIC BEATS:** _____ (present or absent) _____ (unifocal or multifocal) _____ (frequent or infrequent) _____ (R on T).
Conclusion: _____

_____

ANALYSIS

RATE: 75-85/min. (normal). **RHYTHM:** irregular and supraventricular. **P-R INTERVAL:** 0.33 sec. (too long). **QRS DURATION:** 0.10 sec. (normal). **Q-T INTERVAL:** varies (too short). **P' WAVES:** absent. **JUNCTIONAL ECTOPIC BEATS:** absent. **VENTRICULAR ECTOPIC BEATS:** absent. **Conclusion:** Because the P-R interval is so long in this tracing, it almost looks as if the P wave belongs to the preceding QRS. However, the slight sinus arrhythmia shows us that the P wave has a constant relationship to the following ventricular complex. This is unmistakably a first-degree heart block.

EXERCISE 5-2

II

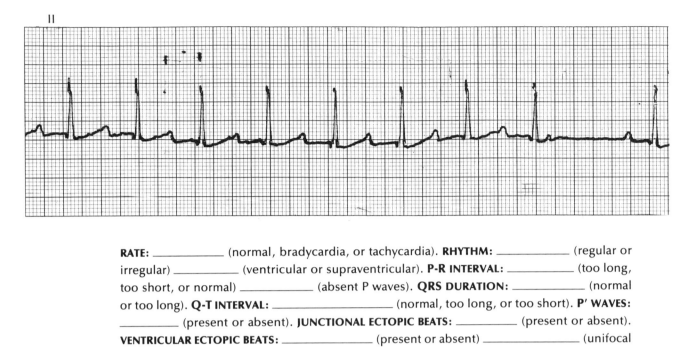

RATE: _____ (normal, bradycardia, or tachycardia). **RHYTHM:** _____ (regular or irregular) _____ (ventricular or supraventricular). **P-R INTERVAL:** _____ (too long, too short, or normal) _____ (absent P waves). **QRS DURATION:** _____ (normal or too long). **Q-T INTERVAL:** _____ (normal, too long, or too short). **P' WAVES:** _____ (present or absent). **JUNCTIONAL ECTOPIC BEATS:** _____ (present or absent). **VENTRICULAR ECTOPIC BEATS:** _____ (present or absent) _____ (unifocal or multifocal) _____ (frequent or infrequent) _____ (R on T). **Conclusion:** _____

_____

ANALYSIS

RATE: 85/min. (normal). **RHYTHM:** irregular and supraventricular. **P-R INTERVAL:** 0.32 sec. (too long). **QRS DURATION:** 0.08 sec. (normal). **Q-T INTERVAL:** difficult to determine. **P' WAVES:** present. **JUNCTIONAL ECTOPIC BEATS:** present and escape. **VENTRICULAR ECTOPIC BEATS:** absent.

Conclusion: Here is a first-degree heart block with marked lengthening of the P-R interval. The rhythm is abruptly interrupted by a nonconducted PAC, which distorts the T wave before the pause. The P wave after the pause may or may not be conducted. It has a shorter P-R interval than the others and may therefore represent a junctional escape beat or a latent Wenckebach.

As you examine this tracing and the preceding one, keep in mind that when a P wave falls midway between two R waves, there is a chance that there is a hidden P' wave and that the rhythm is really an atrial tachycardia with 2:1 block. Carefully examine the QRS-T for any signs of distortion. In this case the nonconducted P' wave seen interrupting the sinus rhythm rules out this possibility.

EXERCISE 5-3

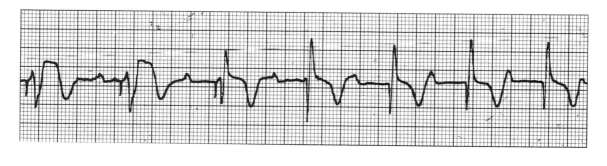

RATE: _____ (normal, bradycardia, or tachycardia). **RHYTHM:** _____ (regular or irregular) _____ (ventricular or supraventricular). **P-R INTERVAL:** _____ (too long, too short, or normal) _____ (absent P waves). **QRS DURATION:** _____ (normal or too long). **Q-T INTERVAL:** _____ (normal, too long, or too short). **P' WAVES:** _____ (present or absent). **JUNCTIONAL ECTOPIC BEATS:** _____ (present or absent). **VENTRICULAR ECTOPIC BEATS:** _____ (present or absent) _____ (unifocal or multifocal) _____ (frequent or infrequent) _____ (R on T).
Conclusion: _____
_____

ANALYSIS

RATE: 60/min. (pacemaker). **RHYTHM:** pacemaker and sinus. **P-R INTERVAL:** 0.38 sec. (too long). **QRS DURATION:** 0.10 (normal). **Q-T INTERVAL:** 0.42 sec. (too long). **P' WAVES:** absent. **JUNCTIONAL ECTOPIC BEATS:** absent. **VENTRICULAR ECTOPIC BEATS:** absent.

Conclusion: The pacemaker spike at the beginning of this tracing is easily seen as a negative spike just preceding the broad ventricular complex. This is a demand pacemaker set at a rate of 60/min. After the third pacemaker spike you will notice a ventricular complex that is unlike the other pacemaker-induced complexes and yet narrower and of lesser amplitude than the sinus-conducted beats that follow. It is a ventricular fusion beat (in this case, pacemaker fusion) caused by the simultaneous activation of the ventricles by two separate wave fronts, one conducted from the sinus node and the other from the pacemaker electrode. Then follows a sinus rhythm with first-degree A-V heart block.

EXERCISE 5-4

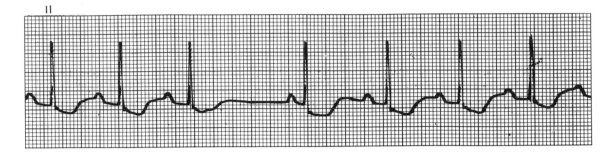

II

RATE: _____ _____ (normal, bradycardia, or tachycardia). **RHYTHM:** _____ (regular or irregular) _____ (ventricular or supraventricular). **P-R INTERVAL:** _____ (too long, too short, or normal) _____ (absent P waves). **QRS DURATION:** _____ (normal or too long). **Q-T INTERVAL:** _____ (normal, too long, or too short). **P′ WAVES:** _____ (present or absent). **JUNCTIONAL ECTOPIC BEATS:** _____ (present or absent). **VENTRICULAR ECTOPIC BEATS:** _____ (present or absent) _____ (unifocal or multifocal) _____ (frequent or infrequent) _____ (R on T).

Conclusion: _____

_____

ANALYSIS

RATE: 80/min. (normal). **RHYTHM:** irregular and supraventricular. **P-R INTERVAL:** 0.24 sec. (too long). **QRS DURATION:** 0.06 sec. (normal). **Q-T INTERVAL:** 0.36 sec. (normal). **P′ WAVES:** absent. **JUNCTIONAL ECTOPIC BEATS:** present and escape. **VENTRICULAR ECTOPIC BEATS:** absent.

Conclusion: This tracing represents first-degree heart block with a nonconducted PAC followed by an escape atrial complex. The arrhythmia looks like sinus exit block (sinus arrest); however, on close examination, the S-T segment just preceding the pause is found to have a little hump in it. When you compare this S-T segment with the two preceding ones, you will easily see the P′ wave, which is not conducted because it is so premature that the A-V junction is still refractory.

Here, as in exercise 5-2, the P-R interval following the pause is shorter than all of the others, and the same possibilities exist; a junctional escape beat fires before the P wave can conduct or Wenckebach conduction.

EXERCISE 5-5

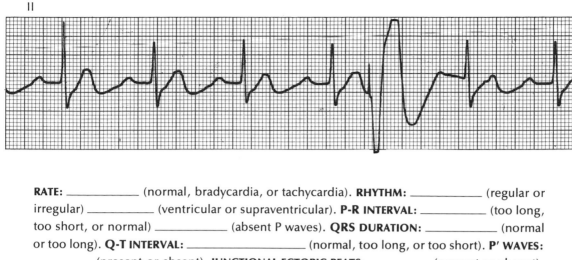

II

RATE: _____ (normal, bradycardia, or tachycardia). **RHYTHM:** _____ (regular or irregular) _____ (ventricular or supraventricular). **P-R INTERVAL:** _____ (too long, too short, or normal) _____ (absent P waves). **QRS DURATION:** _____ (normal or too long). **Q-T INTERVAL:** _____ (normal, too long, or too short). **P′ WAVES:** _____ (present or absent). **JUNCTIONAL ECTOPIC BEATS:** _____ (present or absent). **VENTRICULAR ECTOPIC BEATS:** _____ (present or absent) _____ (unifocal or multifocal) _____ (frequent or infrequent) _____ (R on T).

Conclusion: _____

_____

ANALYSIS

RATE: 62/min. (normal). **RHYTHM:** irregular and supraventricular. **P-R INTERVAL:** 0.28 sec. (too long; constant). **QRS DURATION:** 0.10 sec. (normal). **Q-T INTERVAL:** 0.40 sec. (normal). **P′ WAVES:** absent. **JUNCTIONAL ECTOPIC BEATS:** absent. **VENTRICULAR ECTOPIC BEATS:** absent.

Conclusion: This tracing shows a pacemaker malfunction. The demand pacemaker has obviously been set to fire at a rate slower than the patient's present sinus rhythm. Yet there is a pacemaker spike seen in the first R wave and later on in the strip after a T wave. This malfunction should be corrected, since not only does such random firing compete with the patient's rhythm but also there is a danger that it will fire during the vulnerable period and cause a serious arrhythmia. The underlying rhythm here is that of a first-degree A-V block.

EXERCISE 5-6

II

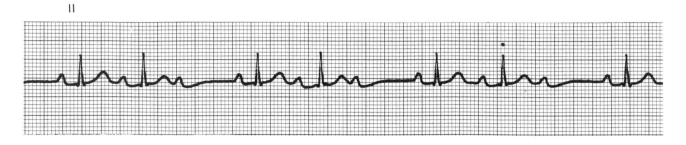

RATE: _____ (normal, bradycardia, or tachycardia). **RHYTHM:** _____ (regular or irregular) _____ (ventricular or supraventricular). **P-R INTERVAL:** _____ (too long, too short, or normal) _____ (absent P waves). **QRS DURATION:** _____ (normal or too long). **Q-T INTERVAL:** _____ (normal, too long, or too short). **P′ WAVES:** _____ (present or absent). **JUNCTIONAL ECTOPIC BEATS:** _____ (present or absent). **VENTRICULAR ECTOPIC BEATS:** _____ (present or absent) _____ (unifocal or multifocal) _____ (frequent or infrequent) _____ (R on T).
Conclusion: _____
_____

ANALYSIS

RATE: approximately 70/min. (normal). **RHYTHM:** irregular and supraventricular. **P-R INTERVAL:** 0.20 and 0.23 sec. (too long; varies). **QRS DURATION:** 0.09 sec. **P′ WAVES:** absent. **JUNCTIONAL ECTOPIC BEATS:** absent. **VENTRICULAR ECTOPIC BEATS:** absent.

Conclusion: This is a second-degree heart block with Wenckebach conduction (type I). The conduction ratio is 3:2. Notice the group beating in this tracing. This is one of the signs that should alert you to Wenckebach. Very often this arrhythmia presents a very confusing picture because the pause and lengthening P-R intervals make it appear that the sinus rhythm is irregular. If you walk out the P waves, you will find them to be right on time.

EXERCISE 5-7

V₁

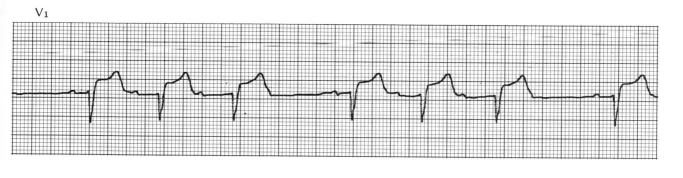

RATE: _____ (normal, bradycardia, or tachycardia). **RHYTHM:** _____ (regular or irregular) _____ (ventricular or supraventricular). **P-R INTERVAL:** _____ (too long, too short, or normal) _____ (absent P waves). **QRS DURATION:** _____ (normal or too long). **Q-T INTERVAL:** _____ (normal, too long, or too short). **P' WAVES:** _____ (present or absent). **JUNCTIONAL ECTOPIC BEATS:** _____ (present or absent). **VENTRICULAR ECTOPIC BEATS:** _____ (present or absent) _____ (unifocal or multifocal) _____ (frequent or infrequent) _____ (R on T).
Conclusion: _____
_____

ANALYSIS

RATE: 65-70/min. (normal). **RHYTHM:** irregular and supraventricular. **P-R INTERVAL:** 0.18, 0.26, and 0.36 sec. (too long; varies). **QRS DURATION:** 0.09 sec. **P' WAVES:** absent. **JUNCTIONAL ECTOPIC BEATS:** absent. **VENTRICULAR ECTOPIC BEATS:** absent.

Conclusion: Here again is the group beating that is so characteristic of Wenckebach. This is second-degree heart block, type I. This time the conduction ratio is 4:3, that is, for every four P waves, three of them are conducted. If you start at the beginning of the tracing and walk out the P waves, you will find the fourth P wave of each set (right on time) distorting the third T wave of that set.

EXERCISE 5-8

III

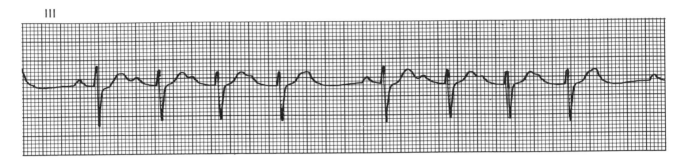

RATE: _____ (normal, bradycardia, or tachycardia). **RHYTHM:** _____ (regular or irregular) _____ (ventricular or supraventricular). **P-R INTERVAL:** _____ (too long, too short, or normal) _____ (absent P waves). **QRS DURATION:** _____ (normal or too long). **Q-T INTERVAL:** _____ (normal, too long, or too short). **P′ WAVES:** _____ (present or absent). **JUNCTIONAL ECTOPIC BEATS:** _____ (present or absent). **VENTRICULAR ECTOPIC BEATS:** _____ (present or absent) _____ (unifocal or multifocal) _____ (frequent or infrequent) _____ (R on T).

Conclusion: _____

ANALYSIS

RATE: approximately 80/min. (normal). **RHYTHM:** irregular and supraventricular. **P-R INTERVAL:** 0.20, 0.26, 0.28, and 0.32 sec. (too long; varies). **QRS DURATION:** 0.09 sec. (normal). **Q-T INTERVAL:** varies (normal). **P′ WAVES:** absent. **JUNCTIONAL ECTOPIC BEATS:** absent. **VENTRICULAR ECTOPIC BEATS:** absent.

Conclusion: This is Wenckebach 5:4. The P waves are not as easily seen in this tracing. However, group beating will alert you to the possibility of Wenckebach conduction. The first two P waves are noticeable. If you walk them out, you will find all of the others on time and distorting T waves.

When the diagnosis to an arrhythmia is not immediately self-evident, maintain a standard approach. First, what is the sinus node doing? Second, establish whether or not there is A-V conduction. An irregular rhythm indicates some conduction since an idioventricular or idiojunctional rhythm would be absolutely regular. Finally, measure the P-Rs. In this case you cannot help but come up with the diagnosis of lengthening P-R intervals and dropped beats (Wenckebach).

EXERCISE 5-9

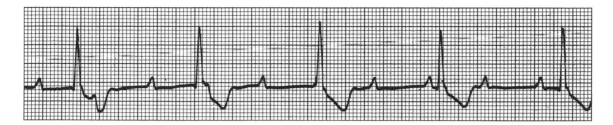

RATE: _____ (normal, bradycardia, or tachycardia). **RHYTHM:** _____ (regular or irregular) _____ (ventricular or supraventricular). **P-R INTERVAL:** _____ (too long, too short, or normal) _____ (absent P waves). **QRS DURATION:** _____ (normal or too long). **Q-T INTERVAL:** _____ (normal, too long, or too short). **P' WAVES:** _____ (present or absent). **JUNCTIONAL ECTOPIC BEATS:** _____ (present or absent). **VENTRICULAR ECTOPIC BEATS:** _____ (present or absent) _____ (unifocal or multifocal) _____ (frequent or infrequent) _____ (R on T).
Conclusion: _____
_____

ANALYSIS

RATE: 46/min., ventricular (bradycardia). RHYTHM: regular and supraventricular. P-R INTERVAL: not applicable. QRS DURATION: 0.08 sec. (normal). Q-T INTERVAL: 0.46 sec. (normal). P' WAVES: absent. JUNCTIONAL ECTOPIC BEATS: present and escape. VENTRICULAR ECTOPIC BEATS: absent.

Conclusion: Did you fall into the trap of calling this a second-degree heart block with 2:1 A-V conduction? Whenever you make such a diagnosis, follow it up by making sure that all of the P-R intervals are the same. In this case they are not. This is a complete, or third-degree, A-V heart block with an idiojunctional rhythm. The ventricular rate is 46/min., and the atrial rate is 100/min. An idiojunctional rhythm is distinguished from an idioventricular rhythm by the duration of the QRS complex. If the ventricles are paced by the A-V junction, the QRS will be normal. If the pacemaker is below the branching portion of the bundle of His, the QRS will be broad and the rate will be slower and less dependable than an idiojunctional pacemaker. In this arrhythmia the atria and the ventricles beat entirely independently of each other, which means that some of the R waves may be superimposed on a P wave. In this tracing all the P waves except one are visible. There is one distorting the first and second S-T segments and one hidden by the third R wave.

EXERCISE 5-10

II

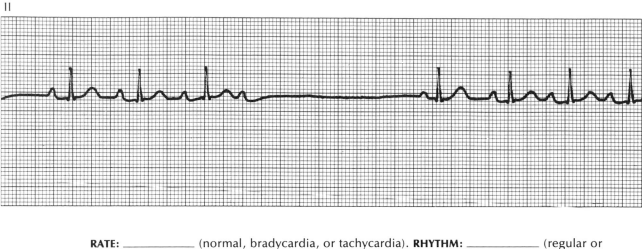

RATE: _____ (normal, bradycardia, or tachycardia). **RHYTHM:** _____ (regular or irregular) _____ (ventricular or supraventricular). **P-R INTERVAL:** _____ (too long, too short, or normal) _____ (absent P waves). **QRS DURATION:** _____ (normal or too long). **Q-T INTERVAL:** _____ (normal, too long, or too short). **P′ WAVES:** _____ (present or absent). **JUNCTIONAL ECTOPIC BEATS:** _____ (present or absent). **VENTRICULAR ECTOPIC BEATS:** _____ (present or absent) _____ (unifocal or multifocal) _____ (frequent or infrequent) _____ (R on T).
Conclusion: _____
_____

ANALYSIS

RATE: approximately 60/min. (normal). **RHYTHM:** irregular and supraventricular. **P-R INTERVAL:** 0.20, 0.23, and 0.25 sec. (too long and varies). **QRS DURATION:** 0.09 sec. (normal). **Q-T INTERVAL:** varies. **P′ WAVES:** absent. **JUNCTIONAL ECTOPIC BEATS:** absent. **VENTRICULAR ECTOPIC BEATS:** absent.

Conclusion: This is a type I (Wenckebach) second-degree A-V block with a sinus exit block. You will probably recognize that this tracing is from the same patient as the one in exercise 5-6. However, now there is an additional problem—sinus exit block. You will notice that the P-P intervals are shortening before the long pause. This indicates a Wenckebach of the sinus node as well. The shortening occurs because the largest increment in conduction from the sinus node to the atrial tissue is between the first and second P waves of the group. The typical Wenckebach, whether it is from the sinus node or the A-V node, will have shortening R-R intervals. It should be noted, however, that not all Wenckebachs are typical.

EXERCISE 5-11

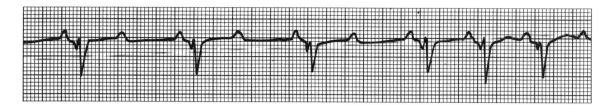

RATE: _____ (normal, bradycardia, or tachycardia). **RHYTHM:** _____ (regular or irregular) _____ (ventricular or supraventricular). **P-R INTERVAL:** _____ (too long, too short, or normal) _____ (absent P waves). **QRS DURATION:** _____ (normal or too long). **Q-T INTERVAL:** _____ (normal, too long, or too short). **P' WAVES:** _____ (present or absent). **JUNCTIONAL ECTOPIC BEATS:** _____ (present or absent). **VENTRICULAR ECTOPIC BEATS:** _____ (present or absent) _____ (unifocal or multifocal) _____ (frequent or infrequent) _____ (R on T).
Conclusion: _____
_____

ANALYSIS

RATE: 48-96/min. (bradycardia to normal). **RHYTHM:** irregular and supraventricular. **P-R INTERVAL:** 0.14 sec. (normal; constant). **QRS DURATION:** 0.14 sec. (too long). **Q-T INTERVAL:** impossible to determine. **P' WAVES:** absent. **JUNCTIONAL ECTOPIC BEATS:** absent. **VENTRICULAR ECTOPIC BEATS:** absent.

Conclusion: This is a type II second-degree A-V block. The last part of the tracing gives an opportunity to see two or more conducted beats in a row and thus rule out type I, or Wenckebach. This type of A-V block is usually accompanied by a broad QRS complex, since the lesion is at the branching portion of the bundle of His. Type II A-V block is associated with a less favorable prognosis than is the Wenckebach type and almost always requires a pacemaker.

EXERCISE 5-12

RATE: _____ (normal, bradycardia, or tachycardia). **RHYTHM:** _____ (regular or irregular) _____ (ventricular or supraventricular). **P-R INTERVAL:** _____ (too long, too short, or normal) _____ (absent P waves). **QRS DURATION:** _____ (normal or too long). **Q-T INTERVAL:** _____ (normal, too long, or too short). **P' WAVES:** _____ (present or absent). **JUNCTIONAL ECTOPIC BEATS:** _____ (present or absent). **VENTRICULAR ECTOPIC BEATS:** _____ ___ (present or absent) _____ (unifocal or multifocal) _____ (frequent or infrequent) _____ (R on T). **Conclusion:** _____ _____

ANALYSIS

RATE: 47/min., ventricular (bradycardia). RHYTHM: irregular and supraventricular. P-R INTERVAL: 0.20 and 0.30 sec. (too long; inconstant). QRS DURATION: 0.10 (normal). Q-T INTERVAL: 0.44 sec. (normal). P' WAVES: absent. JUNCTIONAL ECTOPIC BEATS: absent. VENTRICULAR ECTOPIC BEATS: absent.

Conclusion: This is second-degree A-V block, type I. The beginning of this tracing shows 2:1 A-V conduction (that is, two P waves for every QRS complex) and a P-R interval of 0.20 sec. However, if you look at the group of complexes at the end of the strip, you will see that there is a P-R interval of 0.20 sec., followed by another conducted P wave with a P-R interval of 0.30 sec., and then a P wave (on the T) that is not conducted. This lengthening of the P-R interval with a nonconducted beat constitutes type I (Wenckebach) second-degree A-V block. When there are three P waves for two ventricular complexes, it is called a 3:2 conduction. As long as there are two conducted P waves in a row, you will have no difficulty in diagnosing the type of block. However, when there is 2:1 conduction (every other P wave) it becomes impossible to differentiate between type I and type II second-degree heart block. The duration of the QRS complex can be of some help to you in this dilemma. It has been shown that type I is a function of the A-V node. The lengthening P-R intervals would then be accompanied by a narrow QRS complex. Type II almost always involves a lesion lower in the conductive system, at the branching portion of the bundle of His, and hence is accompanied by a broad QRS complex. In this tracing, if you did not have the two conducted P waves in a row to go by, the narrow QRS would favor type I.

EXERCISE 5-13

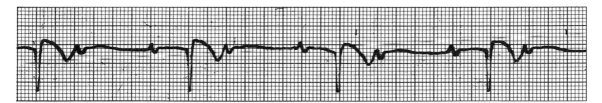

RATE: _____ (normal, bradycardia, or tachycardia). **RHYTHM:** _____ (regular or irregular) _____ (ventricular or supraventricular). **P-R INTERVAL:** _____ (too long, too short, or normal) _____ (absent P waves). **QRS DURATION:** _____ (normal or too long). **Q-T INTERVAL:** _____ (normal, too long, or too short). **P' WAVES:** _____ (present or absent). **JUNCTIONAL ECTOPIC BEATS:** _____ (present or absent). **VENTRICULAR ECTOPIC BEATS:** _____ (present or absent) _____ (unifocal or multifocal) _____ (frequent or infrequent) _____ (R on T).
Conclusion: _____
_____

ANALYSIS

RATE: 37/min. (bradycardia). **RHYTHM:** regular and supraventricular. **P-R INTERVAL:** 0.40 sec. (too long; constant). **QRS DURATION:** 0.08 sec. (normal). **Q-T INTERVAL:** difficult to determine. **P' WAVES:** absent. **JUNCTIONAL ECTOPIC BEATS:** absent. **VENTRICULAR ECTOPIC BEATS:** absent.

Conclusion: This is a second-degree A-V heart block, probably type I, with 2:1 A-V conduction. Since there are not two conducted beats in a row, we are unable to determine whether the P-R interval is lengthened or not. However, since the QRS duration is normal, we know that the block is above the branching portion of the bundle of His and can therefore assume that this is a partial block of the A-V node (Wenckebach).

EXERCISE 5-14

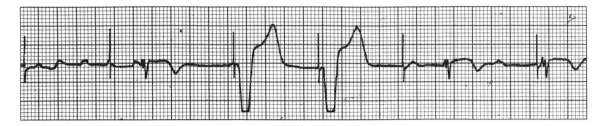

RATE: _____ (normal, bradycardia, or tachycardia). **RHYTHM:** _____ (regular or irregular) _____ (ventricular or supraventricular). **P-R INTERVAL:** _____ (too long, too short, or normal) _____ _____ (absent P waves). **QRS DURATION:** _____ (normal or too long). **Q-T INTERVAL:** _____ (normal, too long, or too short). **P' WAVES:** _____ (present or absent). **JUNCTIONAL ECTOPIC BEATS:** _____ (present or absent).

VENTRICULAR ECTOPIC BEATS: _____ (present or absent) _____ (unifocal or multifocal) _____ (frequent or infrequent) _____ (R on T).

Conclusion: _____

_____

ANALYSIS

RATE: 50/min. (bradycardia). RHYTHM: malfunctioning pacemaker and irregular supraventricular. **P-R INTERVAL:** 0.36, 0.48, and 0.58 sec. (too long; constant). **QRS DURATION:** 0.08 sec. (normal). **Q-T INTERVAL:** 0.46 sec. (normal). **P' WAVES:** absent. **JUNCTIONAL ECTOPIC BEATS:** absent. **VENTRICULAR ECTOPIC BEATS:** absent.

Conclusion: This is a malfunctioning demand pacemaker. The demand mode is functioning properly; that is, the pacemaker is sensing ventricular complexes and resetting itself to fire at its preset interval. However, there are only two capture beats in the strip, which are noticeable in the middle of the tracing. The failure of this pacemaker to capture, or depolarize, the ventricles results in the dominance of the patient's own rhythm, which is a type I second-degree A-V heart block with a short burst of atrial tachycardia (nonconducted) at the beginning of the tracing.

EXERCISE 5-15

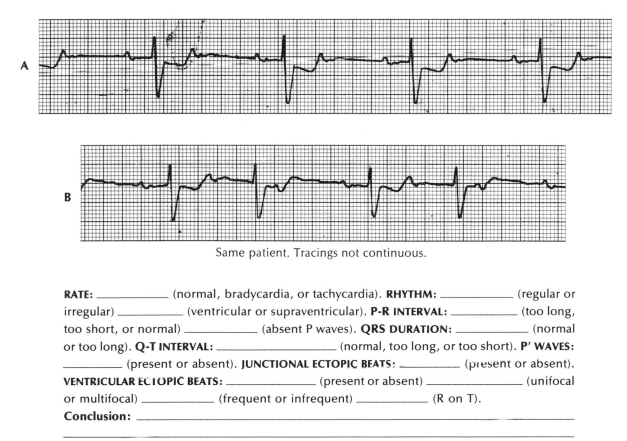

Same patient. Tracings not continuous.

RATE: _____ (normal, bradycardia, or tachycardia). **RHYTHM:** _____ (regular or irregular) _____ (ventricular or supraventricular). **P-R INTERVAL:** _____ (too long, too short, or normal) _____ (absent P waves). **QRS DURATION:** _____ (normal or too long). **Q-T INTERVAL:** _____ (normal, too long, or too short). **P' WAVES:** _____ (present or absent). **JUNCTIONAL ECTOPIC BEATS:** _____ (present or absent). **VENTRICULAR ECTOPIC BEATS:** _____ (present or absent) _____ (unifocal or multifocal) _____ (frequent or infrequent) _____ (R on T). **Conclusion:** _____

ANALYSIS

RATE: 43-66/min. (bradycardia to normal). RHYTHM: A, regular; B, irregular; supraventricular in both. P-R INTERVAL: A, 0.28 sec. (constant; too long); B, 0.32 and 0.44 sec. (inconstant; too long). QRS DURATION: 0.13 sec. (too long). Q-T INTERVAL: difficult to determine. P' WAVES: absent. JUNCTIONAL ECTOPIC BEATS: absent. VENTRICULAR ECTOPIC BEATS: absent.

Conclusion: This is a type I second-degree A-V block. In the second tracing, which is from the same patient, two consecutive conducted beats are seen with P-R intervals lengthening from 0.32 to 0.44 sec. The third P wave is then not conducted, constituting a Wenckebach phenomenon. If only the first tracing were available, you would be quite justified in presuming this to be a type II A-V block, since the QRS duration is prolonged. This lengthening, in addition to the long P-R interval, would cause you to anticipate more serious conduction disturbances, since the lesion probably involves more than one area of the conductive system—the A-V node and the bundle branches.

EXERCISE 5-16

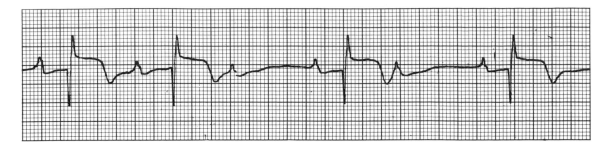

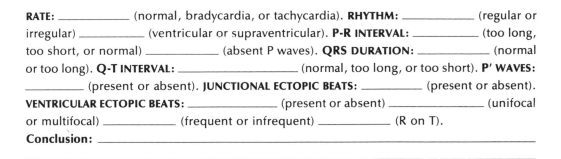

RATE: _____ (normal, bradycardia, or tachycardia). **RHYTHM:** _____ (regular or irregular) _____ (ventricular or supraventricular). **P-R INTERVAL:** _____ (too long, too short, or normal) _____ (absent P waves). **QRS DURATION:** _____ (normal or too long). **Q-T INTERVAL:** _____ (normal, too long, or too short). **P′ WAVES:** _____ (present or absent). **JUNCTIONAL ECTOPIC BEATS:** _____ (present or absent). **VENTRICULAR ECTOPIC BEATS:** _____ (present or absent) _____ (unifocal or multifocal) _____ (frequent or infrequent) _____ (R on T). **Conclusion:** _____
_____

ANALYSIS

RATE: approximately 45/min. (bradycardia). **RHYTHM:** irregular and supraventricular. **P-R INTERVAL:** 0.36 and 0.42 (inconstant; too long). **QRS DURATION:** 0.10 sec. (normal). **Q-T INTERVAL:** 0.58 sec. (too long). **P′ WAVES:** absent. **JUNCTIONAL ECTOPIC BEATS:** absent. **VENTRICULAR ECTOPIC BEATS:** absent.

Conclusion: This is a second-degree A-V block, type I (Wenckebach), with 3.2 and 2:1 A-V conduction. The sinus P waves occur at regular intervals. The P-R interval lengthens, and there are nonconducted beats.

EXERCISE 5-17

II

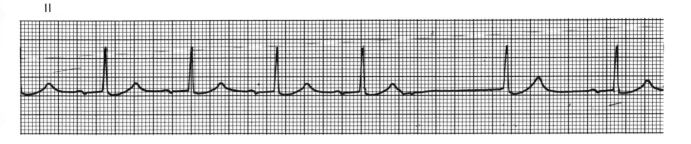

RATE: _____ (normal, bradycardia, or tachycardia). **RHYTHM:** _____ (regular or irregular) _____ (ventricular or supraventricular). **P-R INTERVAL:** _____ (too long, too short, or normal) _____ (absent P waves). **QRS DURATION:** _____ (normal or too long). **Q-T INTERVAL:** _____ (normal, too long, or too short). **P' WAVES:** _____ (present or absent). **JUNCTIONAL ECTOPIC BEATS:** _____ (present or absent). **VENTRICULAR ECTOPIC BEATS:** _____ (present or absent) _____ (unifocal or multifocal) _____ (frequent or infrequent) _____ (R on T).

Conclusion: _____

_____

ANALYSIS

RATE: 60-65/min. (normal). RHYTHM: irregular and supraventricular. P-R INTERVAL: 0.27 sec. (too long). QRS DURATION: 0.08 sec. (normal). Q-T INTERVAL: 0.40 sec. (normal). P' WAVES: present. JUNCTIONAL ECTOPIC BEATS: present. VENTRICULAR ECTOPIC BEATS: absent.

Conclusion: This is a first-degree heart block with a nonconducted PAC, followed by a junctional escape beat. There is a P' wave distorting the T preceding the pause.

EXERCISE 5-18

II

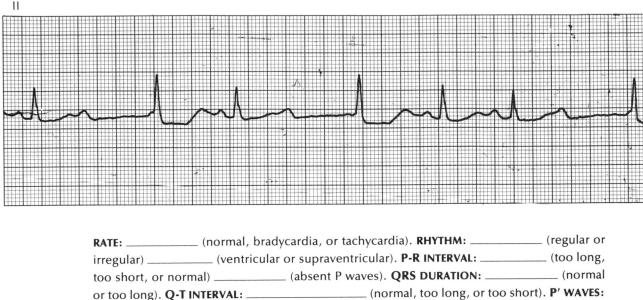

RATE: _____ (normal, bradycardia, or tachycardia). **RHYTHM:** _____ (regular or irregular) _____ (ventricular or supraventricular). **P-R INTERVAL:** _____ (too long, too short, or normal) _____ (absent P waves). **QRS DURATION:** _____ (normal or too long). **Q-T INTERVAL:** _____ (normal, too long, or too short). **P' WAVES:** _____ (present or absent). **JUNCTIONAL ECTOPIC BEATS:** _____ (present or absent). **VENTRICULAR ECTOPIC BEATS:** _____ (present or absent) _____ (unifocal or multifocal) _____ (frequent or infrequent) _____ (R on T). **Conclusion:** _____

_____

ANALYSIS

RATE: 55-60/min. (bradycardia). **RHYTHM:** irregular and supraventricular. **P-R INTERVAL:** 0.18 and 0.20 sec. (varies). **QRS DURATION:** 0.08 sec. (normal). **Q-T INTERVAL:** varies (too long). **P' WAVES:** absent. **JUNCTIONAL ECTOPIC BEATS:** present. **VENTRICULAR ECTOPIC BEATS:** absent.

Conclusion: This is a type I second-degree heart block with junctional escape beats. The Wenckebach cycle can be seen toward the end of the tracing where two conducted beats in a row are seen. Note the slightly different morphology of the junctional escape beats. They are taller than the sinus conducted beats; in addition, they are distorted by a sinus P wave that occurs at the same time, causing the complex to look like it has a delta wave.

If your diagnosis was incorrect, review the following steps. Start from the beginning and walk out the P waves. They are right on time, hiding in Rs and Ts. Then begin to establish conduction. Right away you know that there *is* conduction because of the irregularity of the ventricular rhythm. An idiojunctional rhythm would be absolutely regular. Note that three P-Rs are all the same. They are sinus-conducted beats. The two conducted beats in a row at the end of the tracing confirm the diagnosis. The junctional escape beats are easily spotted not only because they follow the long pause but because they are slightly different in morphology.[61,62]

EXERCISE 5-19

II

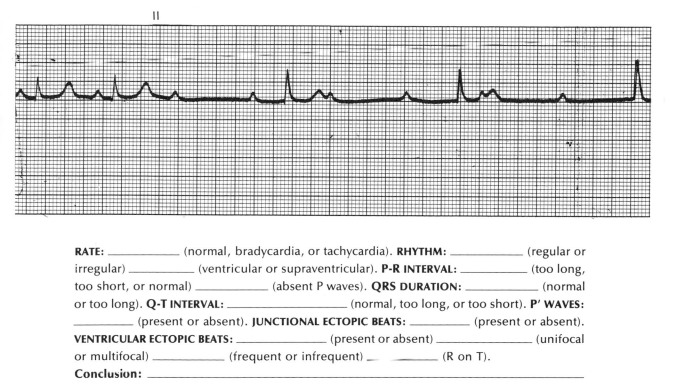

RATE: _____ (normal, bradycardia, or tachycardia). **RHYTHM:** _____ (regular or irregular) _____ (ventricular or supraventricular). **P-R INTERVAL:** _____ (too long, too short, or normal) _____ (absent P waves). **QRS DURATION:** _____ (normal or too long). **Q-T INTERVAL:** _____ (normal, too long, or too short). **P′ WAVES:** _____ (present or absent). **JUNCTIONAL ECTOPIC BEATS:** _____ (present or absent). **VENTRICULAR ECTOPIC BEATS:** _____ (present or absent) _____ (unifocal or multifocal) _____ (frequent or infrequent) _____ (R on T).

Conclusion: _____

_____

ANALYSIS

RATE: 32-40/min. (bradycardia). **RHYTHM:** irregular and supraventricular. **P-R INTERVAL:** 0.20 sec. (too long). **QRS DURATION:** 0.09 sec. (normal). **Q-T INTERVAL:** 0.46 sec. (normal). **P′ WAVES:** absent. **JUNCTIONAL ECTOPIC BEATS:** present. **VENTRICULAR ECTOPIC BEATS:** absent.

Conclusion: Here you see the onset of complete heart block. There is not even an increment in P-R interval preceding the block. The patient is suddenly in third-degree heart block. His heart rate drops from 72-32 beats/min. in a moment. Such an abrupt transition is usually accompanied by Adams-Stokes syndrome.

The escape rhythm accompanying the complete heart block is idiojunctional because the complexes are only slightly different in morphology from the sinus-conducted beats. The last ventricular complex on the tracing is broadened because there is a P wave hidden in it.

You may have said that this patient went into Wenckebach because of the lengthening P-R intervals. Remember that when there are two P waves between R waves, as seen here, all of the P-R intervals have to be exactly the same in order to label it second-degree heart block. When the conduction ratio is 2:1, whether it is Wenckebach or type II second-degree heart block, the P-Rs will all be the same. The P-Rs lengthen in Wenckebach *only when there are two conducted beats in a row.*

EXERCISE 5-20

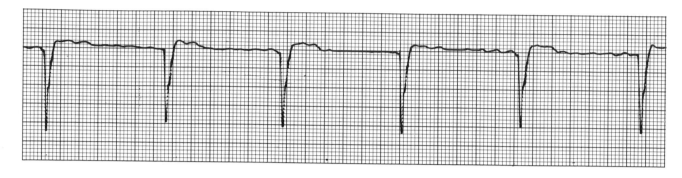

RATE: _____ (normal, bradycardia, or tachycardia). **RHYTHM:** _____ (regular or irregular) _____ (ventricular or supraventricular). **P-R INTERVAL:** _____ (too long, too short, or normal) _____ (absent P waves). **QRS DURATION:** _____ (normal or too long). **Q-T INTERVAL:** _____ (normal, too long, or too short). **P' WAVES:** _____ (present or absent). **JUNCTIONAL ECTOPIC BEATS:** _____ (present or absent).

VENTRICULAR ECTOPIC BEATS: _____ (present or absent) _____ (unifocal or multifocal) _____ (frequent or infrequent) _____ (R on T).

Conclusion: _____

ANALYSIS

RATE: 47/min. (bradycardia). **RHYTHM:** regular and supraventricular. **P-R INTERVAL:** absent P waves. **QRS DURATION:** 0.12 sec. (too long). **Q-T INTERVAL:** difficult to determine. **P' WAVES:** absent. **JUNCTIONAL ECTOPIC BEATS:** present. **VENTRICULAR ECTOPIC BEATS:** absent.

Conclusion: This is atrial fibrillation with complete heart block. The atrial fibrillatory line is seen through the tracing. In atrial fibrillation you expect to encounter an irregular ventricular response. Regularity of the ventricular response indicates that the ventricles are uninfluenced by the erratic atrial activity because there is a block. In such a case there will be either an idiojunctional pacemaker or an idioventricular one. The rate here indicates an idiojunctional pacemaker. However, the QRS is broad, indicating either the presence of BBB or an accelerated idioventricular pacemaker.

Digitalis is given to patients with atrial fibrillation to slow down the ventricular rate, which usually exceeds 100/min. This drug will accomplish this by lengthening the refractory period in the A-V node. If too much digitalis is given, heart block will ensue. You will first note that there is some degree of regularization.[64] Complete block will be manifested by absolute regularity or by group beating, which is discussed in a subsequent exercise.

EXERCISE 5-21

II

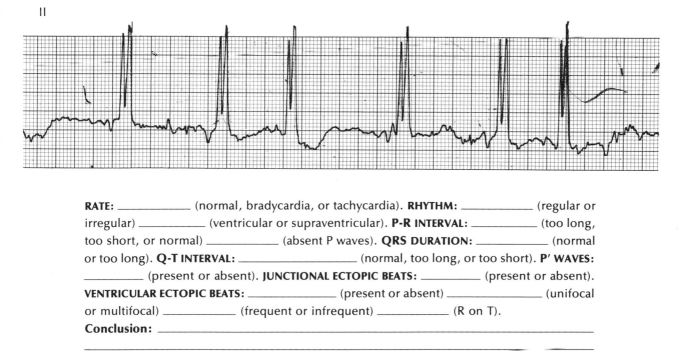

RATE: _____ (normal, bradycardia, or tachycardia). **RHYTHM:** _____ (regular or irregular) _____ (ventricular or supraventricular). **P-R INTERVAL:** _____ (too long, too short, or normal) _____ (absent P waves). **QRS DURATION:** _____ (normal or too long). **Q-T INTERVAL:** _____ (normal, too long, or too short). **P′ WAVES:** _____ (present or absent). **JUNCTIONAL ECTOPIC BEATS:** _____ (present or absent). **VENTRICULAR ECTOPIC BEATS:** _____ (present or absent) _____ (unifocal or multifocal) _____ (frequent or infrequent) _____ (R on T).

Conclusion: _____

ANALYSIS

RATE: approximately 70/min. (normal). **RHYTHM:** irregular and supraventricular. **P-R INTERVAL:** absent P waves. **QRS DURATION:** 0.12 sec. (too long). **Q-T INTERVAL:** difficult to determine. **P′ WAVES:** absent. **JUNCTIONAL ECTOPIC BEATS:** present. **VENTRICULAR ECTOPIC BEATS:** absent.

Conclusion: The underlying atrial fibrillation is unmistakable, and at first the irregular ventricular response seems to be appropriate. However, did you notice group beating? There are two groups of three with shortening R-R intervals and then a pause. This is a sign of Wenckebach. In atrial fibrillation it is another sign of digitalis toxicity.[64] Digitalis in excess may cause a complete heart block, junctional tachycardia, and Wenckebach exit block. In other words, the idiojunctional pacemaker fires at regular intervals (in this case at an accelerated rate); however, the length of time it takes for the impulse to travel from the site of origin to the ventricular tissue lengthens with each beat until one beat is not conducted at all. The cycle then begins all over again.

To review, group beating *and* regularization are both signs of digitalis toxicity in atrial fibrillation.

EXERCISE 5-22

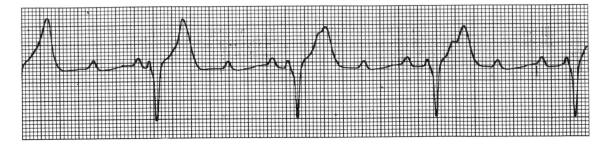

RATE: _____ (normal, bradycardia, or tachycardia). **RHYTHM:** _____ (regular or irregular) _____ (ventricular or supraventricular). **P-R INTERVAL:** _____ (too long, too short, or normal) _____ (absent P waves). **QRS DURATION:** _____ (normal or too long). **Q-T INTERVAL:** _____ (normal, too long, or too short). **P' WAVES:** _____ (present or absent). **JUNCTIONAL ECTOPIC BEATS:** _____ (present or absent).

VENTRICULAR ECTOPIC BEATS: _____ (present or absent) _____ (unifocal or multifocal) _____ (frequent or infrequent) _____ (R on T).

Conclusion: _____

_____

ANALYSIS

RATE: 40/min. (bradycardia). **RHYTHM:** regular and ventricular. **P-R INTERVAL:** not applicable. **QRS DURATION:** 0.16 sec. (too long). **Q-T INTERVAL:** 0.56 sec. (too long). **P' WAVES:** absent. **JUNCTIONAL ECTOPIC BEATS:** absent. **VENTRICULAR ECTOPIC BEATS:** present.

Conclusion: This is a complete heart block with a sinus tachycardia of 125/min. and an idioventricular rate of 40/min. You may think this is type II second-degree heart block. The P-R intervals are, however, all of different lengths, and a closer examination of the T waves reveals hidden P waves. Mark off the first two visible P waves, and walk out the atrial rhythm. You will find the sinus rhythm regular, with P waves hidden in T waves and distorting S-T segments.

EXERCISE 5-23

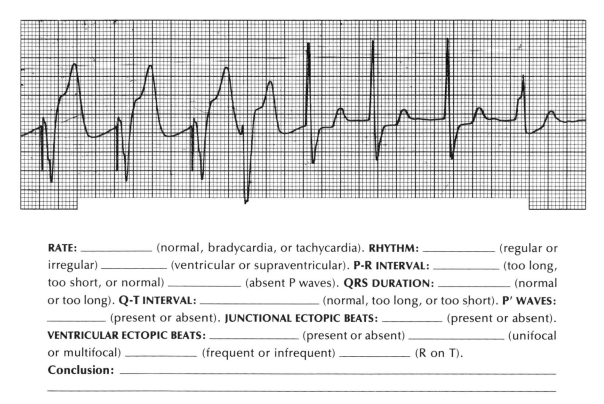

RATE: _____ (normal, bradycardia, or tachycardia). **RHYTHM:** _____ (regular or irregular) _____ (ventricular or supraventricular). **P-R INTERVAL:** _____ (too long, too short, or normal) _____ (absent P waves). **QRS DURATION:** _____ (normal or too long). **Q-T INTERVAL:** _____ (normal, too long, or too short). **P' WAVES:** _____ (present or absent). **JUNCTIONAL ECTOPIC BEATS:** _____ (present or absent). **VENTRICULAR ECTOPIC BEATS:** _____ (present or absent) _____ (unifocal or multifocal) _____ (frequent or infrequent) _____ (R on T).

Conclusion: _____

_____

ANALYSIS

RATE: 75/min. (pacemaker). **RHYTHM:** pacemaker. **P-R INTERVAL:** P waves not seen. **QRS DURATION:** 0.16 sec. (too long). **Q-T INTERVAL:** 0.44 sec. (too long). **P' WAVES:** absent. **JUNCTIONAL ECTOPIC BEATS:** absent. **VENTRICULAR ECTOPIC BEATS:** present, premature, and multifocal.

Conclusion: The first three complexes are a pacemaker-induced rhythm. This is a demand pacemaker set at a rate of 75/min. A demand pacemaker will sense ventricular complexes and will not fire until its own interval is reached. This protects the heart from running in competition with the very instrument that is meant to augment its function. Sometimes the pacemaker spike is not as easy to find as in this strip. It can be very much smaller, especially with a bipolar electrode.

In this tracing the pacemaker rhythm is interrupted by a PVC and therefore does not fire. There are four more complexes after the first PVC, all of which are at a rate faster than the pacemaker's 75/min. and therefore suppress the pacemaker function.

EXERCISE 5-24

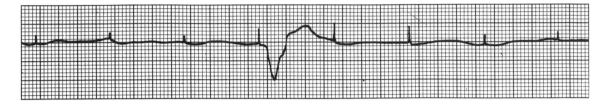

RATE: _____ (normal, bradycardia, or tachycardia). **RHYTHM:** _____ (regular or irregular) _____ (ventricular or supraventricular). **P-R INTERVAL:** _____ (too long, too short, or normal) _____ (absent P waves). **QRS DURATION:** _____ (normal or too long). **Q-T INTERVAL:** _____ _____ (normal, too long, or too short). **P' WAVES:** _____ (present or absent). **JUNCTIONAL ECTOPIC BEATS:** _____ (present or absent).
VENTRICULAR ECTOPIC BEATS: _____ (present or absent) _____ (unifocal or multifocal) _____ (frequent or infrequent) _____ (R on T).
Conclusion: _____

_____

ANALYSIS

RATE: 75/min. (pacemaker).

Conclusion: The pacemaker is firing at a rate of 75/min., but there is only one capture in the 6-inch strip presented here. The amount of electrical energy delivered to the heart may need to be increased; the electrode may need repositioning; or perhaps the heart is incapable of responding.

EXERCISE 5-25

V₁

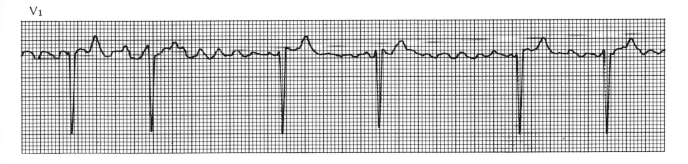

RATE: _____ (normal, bradycardia, or tachycardia). **RHYTHM:** _____ (regular or irregular) _____ (ventricular or supraventricular). **P-R INTERVAL:** _____ (too long, too short, or normal) _____ (absent P waves). **QRS DURATION:** _____ (normal or too long). **Q-T INTERVAL:** _____ (normal, too long, or too short). **P′ WAVES:** _____ (present or absent). **JUNCTIONAL ECTOPIC BEATS:** _____ (present or absent). **VENTRICULAR ECTOPIC BEATS:** _____ (present or absent) _____ (unifocal or multifocal) _____ (frequent or infrequent) _____ (R on T).
Conclusion: _____
_____

ANALYSIS

RATE: 50-60/min. (bradycardia). **RHYTHM:** irregular and supraventricular. **P-R INTERVAL:** absent P waves. **QRS DURATION:** 0.08 sec. (normal). **Q-T INTERVAL:** difficult to determine. **P′ WAVES:** absent. **JUNCTIONAL ECTOPIC BEATS:** present. **VENTRICULAR ECTOPIC BEATS:** absent.

Conclusion: This is atrial fibrillation. As in exercise 5-22, group beating and bradycardia should alert you to the possibility of digitalis excess.

EXERCISE 5-26

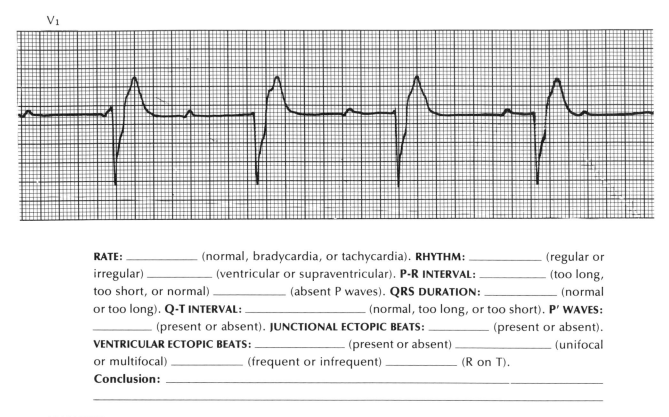

V₁

RATE: _____ (normal, bradycardia, or tachycardia). **RHYTHM:** _____ (regular or irregular) _____ (ventricular or supraventricular). **P-R INTERVAL:** _____ (too long, too short, or normal) _____ (absent P waves). **QRS DURATION:** _____ (normal or too long). **Q-T INTERVAL:** _____ (normal, too long, or too short). **P' WAVES:** _____ (present or absent). **JUNCTIONAL ECTOPIC BEATS:** _____ (present or absent). **VENTRICULAR ECTOPIC BEATS:** _____ (present or absent) _____ (unifocal or multifocal) _____ (frequent or infrequent) _____ (R on T). **Conclusion:** _____

ANALYSIS

RATE: 40/min. (bradycardia). RHYTHM: regular. P-R INTERVAL: not applicable. QRS DURATION: 0.16 sec. (too long). Q-T INTERVAL: 0.40 sec. (too short). P' WAVES: absent. JUNCTIONAL ECTOPIC BEATS: perhaps. VENTRICULAR ECTOPIC BEATS: perhaps.

Conclusion: This is a complete heart block with a sinus rate of approximately 70/min. and a slight sinus arrhythmia. The ventricular rhythm is regular at 40/min. The rate of the ventricular beats may indicate a pacemaker below the branching portion of the bundle of His (broad QRS). An idiojunctional pacemaker with BBB is also a possibility.

Almost every other P wave is hidden in the QRS-T complex. However, the first two P waves are visible and can help you find the others. The second P wave causes the first QRS to look like it begins with a broad r wave.

EXERCISE 5-27

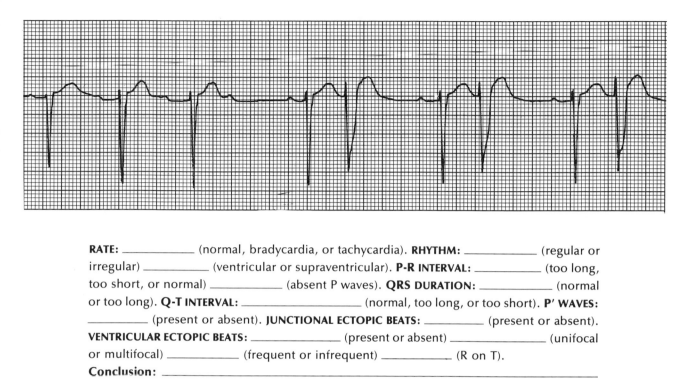

RATE: _____ (normal, bradycardia, or tachycardia). **RHYTHM:** _____ (regular or irregular) _____ (ventricular or supraventricular). **P-R INTERVAL:** _____ (too long, too short, or normal) _____ (absent P waves). **QRS DURATION:** _____ (normal or too long). **Q-T INTERVAL:** _____ (normal, too long, or too short). **P′ WAVES:** _____ (present or absent). **JUNCTIONAL ECTOPIC BEATS:** _____ (present or absent).

VENTRICULAR ECTOPIC BEATS: _____ (present or absent) _____ (unifocal or multifocal) _____ (frequent or infrequent) _____ (R on T).

Conclusion: _____

_____

ANALYSIS

RATE: 80-85/min. (normal). **RHYTHM:** irregular and supraventricular with ventricular. **P-R INTERVAL:** 0.18, 0.24, and 0.30 sec. (too long; varies). **QRS DURATION:** 0.09 sec. (normal). **Q-T INTERVAL:** varies (normal). **P′ WAVES:** absent. **JUNCTIONAL ECTOPIC BEATS:** absent. **VENTRICULAR ECTOPIC BEATS:** present, unifocal, and frequent.

Conclusion: Except for the tell-tale sign at the beginning of this tracing, the bigeminal PVCs would have masked the presence of type I second-degree heart block. Notice the lengthening P-R intervals and the dropped beat (first four P waves).

EXERCISE 5-28

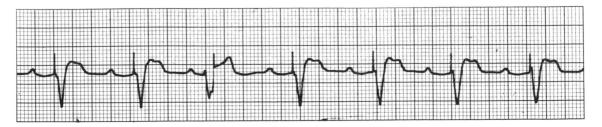

RATE: _____ (normal, bradycardia, or tachycardia). **RHYTHM:** _____ (regular or irregular) _____ (ventricular or supraventricular). **P-R INTERVAL:** _____ (too long, too short, or normal) _____ (absent P waves). **QRS DURATION:** _____ (normal or too long). **Q-T INTERVAL:** _____ (normal, too long, or too short). **P' WAVES:** _____ (present or absent). **JUNCTIONAL ECTOPIC BEATS:** _____ (present or absent). **VENTRICULAR ECTOPIC BEATS:** _____ (present or absent) _____ (unifocal or multifocal) _____ (frequent or infrequent) _____ (R on T).
Conclusion: _____
_____

ANALYSIS

RATE: 70/min. (pacemaker). RHYTHM: irregular.

Conclusion: This tracing represents either a fixed-rate pacemaker or a malfunction of a demand pacemaker. The third complex is sinus conducted with a normal P-R interval, and therefore this complex occurs before the next expected pacemaker discharge. The pacemaker continues its regular rate of 70/min. regardless of the patient's own rhythm. Ventricular depolarization did not occur after this third pacemaker spike because of ventricular refractoriness.

EXERCISE 5-29

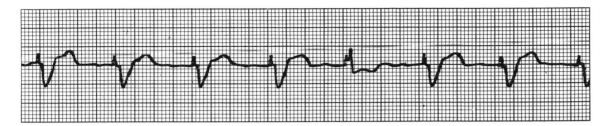

RATE: _____ (normal, bradycardia, or tachycardia). **RHYTHM:** _____ (regular or irregular) _____ (ventricular or supraventricular). **P-R INTERVAL:** _____ (too long, too short, or normal) _____ (absent P waves). **QRS DURATION:** _____ (normal or too long). **Q-T INTERVAL:** _____ (normal, too long, or too short). **P' WAVES:** _____ (present or absent). **JUNCTIONAL ECTOPIC BEATS:** _____ (present or absent). **VENTRICULAR ECTOPIC BEATS:** _____ (present or absent) _____ (unifocal or multifocal) _____ (frequent or infrequent) _____ (R on T).

Conclusion: _____

_____

ANALYSIS

RATE: 72/min. (pacemaker).

Conclusion: This tracing depicts a properly functioning demand pacemaker. The fifth pacemaker spike does not capture, presumably because a ventricular ectopic beat occurs simultaneously.

CHAPTER 6
LADDERGRAMS

Laddergrams are simply graphic displays of the chronological conduction events within the heart. Some of the more complex arrhythmias are best explained by the use of laddergrams. Fig. 1 is designed so that you can visually relate the heart to the sections of the laddergram. The first small section is reserved for the activity of the sinus node and is only used when there is a conduction problem between the sinus node and the atrial tissue.

The laddergram should tell you where the pacemaker for a particular complex originated. This is done by beginning the graph in the section where the impulse had its origin. All lines then proceed from this leading point. The laddergram will also display the speed of conduction of a particular complex. For example, the conduction time through the A-V junction is indicated by a line that begins at the end of the P wave and proceeds downward and forward to the beginning of the ventricular complex. In Fig. 1 several pacemaker and conduction possibilities are shown. When constructing your own laddergram, you should draw the atrial and ventricular lines first, since they are so apparent, and then fill in the A-V junctional activity. In so doing, you may notice some hidden mechanism.

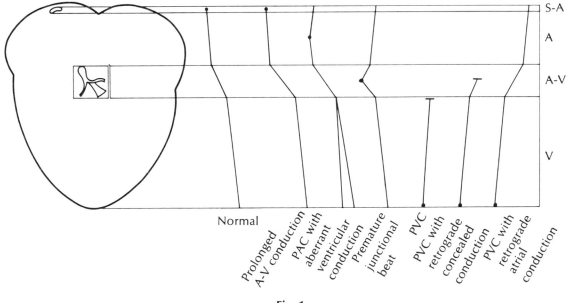

Fig. 1

EXERCISE 6-1

V₁

A

A-V

V

Begin your laddergram by filling in the P waves in the A tier and then the ventricular complexes in the V tier. Compare what you have done with the laddergram below. Notice that since the laddergram depicts a *sequence* of events, the PACs will be indicated by placing a leading point in the middle of the A tier instead of at the top of it as is done for the sinus P waves. Now simply fill in A-V conduction by drawing a straight line from the end of the P wave line to the top of the QRS line.

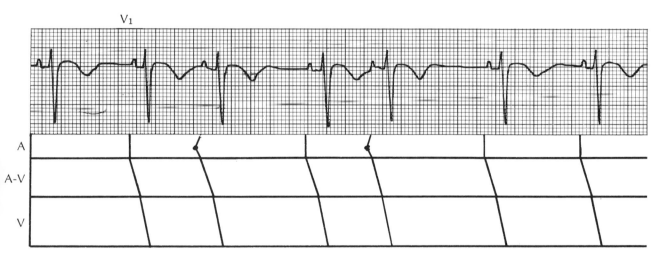

V₁

A

A-V

V

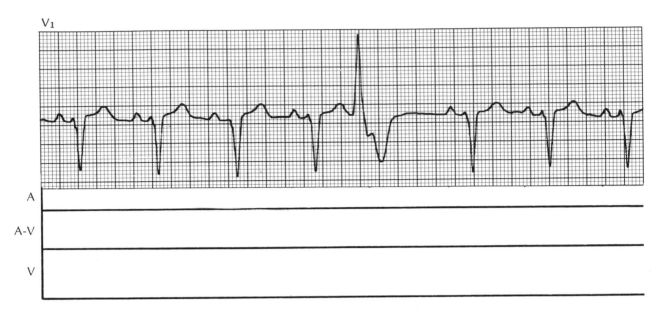

Begin your laddergram as before, and you will easily find the hidden sinus P wave occurring right on time. It is in the T wave of the ectopic beat.

The ventricular ectopic complex is illustrated by placing the leading point at the bottom of the V tier at a spot directly below where the PVC begins. The V line will then proceed upward in this tier, slanted toward the top of the tier at a spot directly below where the PVC ends. Normally conducted ventricular complexes are illustrated this way, too, but the slant is in the opposite direction, that is, beginning at the top of the V tier and ending at the bottom. The V line will give you some idea of intraventricular conduction time because it is slanted.

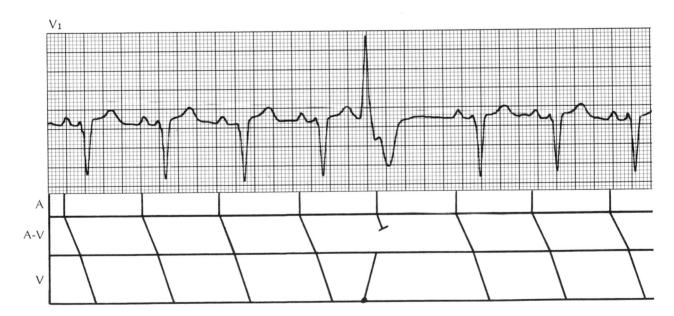

EXERCISE 6-3

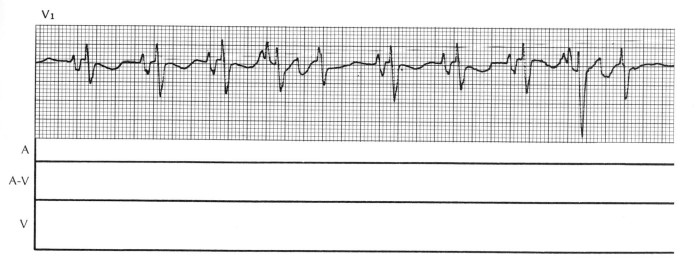

This is a more complicated mechanism to illustrate since there is an atrial echo and a ventricular reciprocal beat. However, the laddergram is the most useful tool to explain this mechanism.

Begin, as before, by marking the P lines in the A tier. Indicate the two PACs that are so evident. Unless you are experienced and aware of reciprocating mechanisms, you will probably not see the atrial echo beat. Just leave it for now, and draw in the ventricular lines in the V tier. Indicate A-V conduction; it is immediately apparent that there is a ventricular complex with no origin. You can find the atrial echo beat in the T wave preceding the complex in question. The PAC has caused dissociation within the A-V node, passing antegradely to capture the ventricles and then retrogradely to recapture the atria and back down again to the ventricles. The laddergram depicts this mechanism well. The PAC at the end of the tracing is conducted with aberrancy.

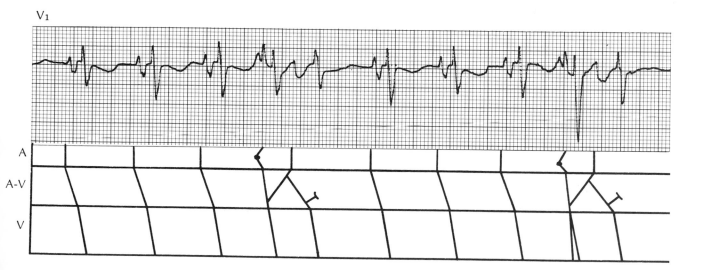

EXERCISE 6-4

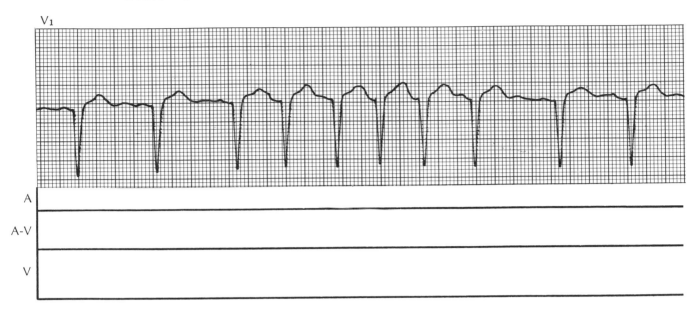

Here is another reciprocating mechanism. See if you can construct the laddergram and then compare yours with the one below.

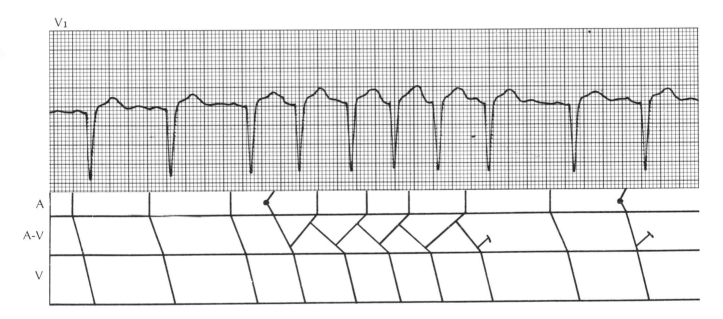

EXERCISE 6-5

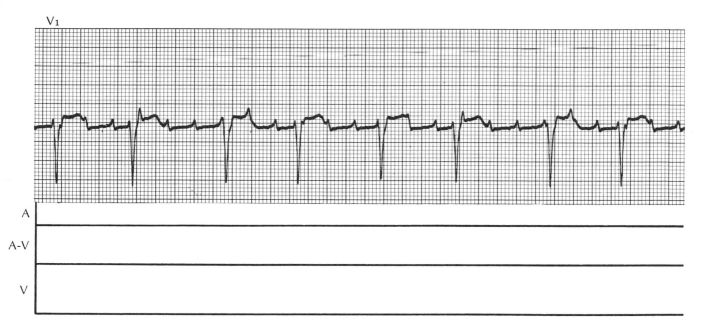

This is atrial flutter as seen in V_1. When the P'-R interval alternates like this, there is a Wenckebach conduction mechanism. Draw in the P' waves. Since all are ectopic, simply draw them as you would sinus P waves. Their rate alone will indicate ectopy. Now draw in the ventricular complexes, and see if you can establish the right A-V conduction lines, keeping in mind a Wenckebach type of conduction. Compare your laddergram with the one below.

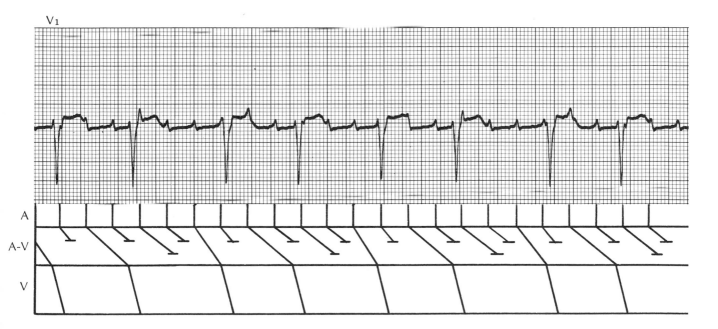

EXERCISE 6-6

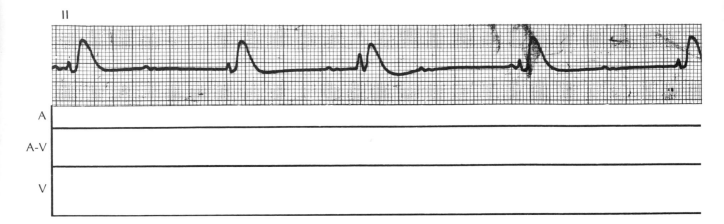

In this exercise mark in the P waves that you see. If you keep in mind the normal behavior of the sinus node, you will find the hidden ones. Draw in the ventricular complexes. They are very low in amplitude with very tall T waves. Draw the A-V conduction lines, remembering the rule that when the P-R intervals are all different, the R-R intervals must all be equal for it to be complete heart block. If there is a QRS out of step, it will be "pulled in" (early, conducted). Compare your laddergram with the one below. This is a high-grade second-degree heart block. Notice that the conducted beat is of slightly different morphology.

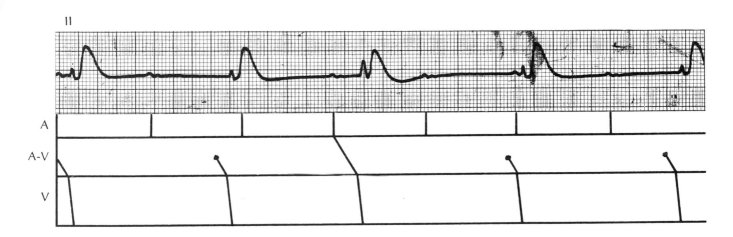

EXERCISE 6-7

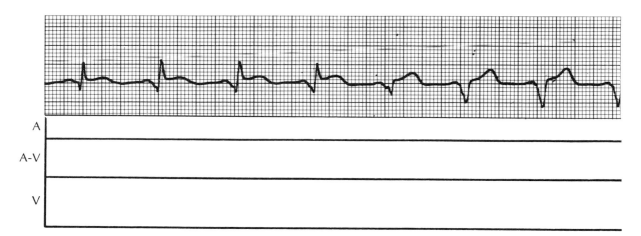

Conclusion: The sinus rate in this tracing is 74/min. There is an accelerated idio-ventricular focus competing at a rate of 75/min. The ventricular ectopic focus can be seen manifesting itself in the second complex. This complex and the four after it are fusion beats, with the ventricular ectopic focus capturing the ventricles more completely each time until finally it is premature enough for complete capture.

The laddergram appropriately illustrates why ventricular fusion beats seldom look just the same in a particular lead. It is because the degrees of fusion are never exactly the same.

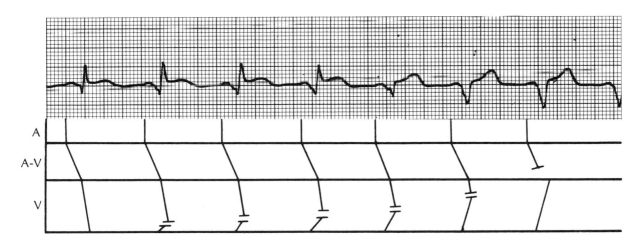

EXERCISE 6-8

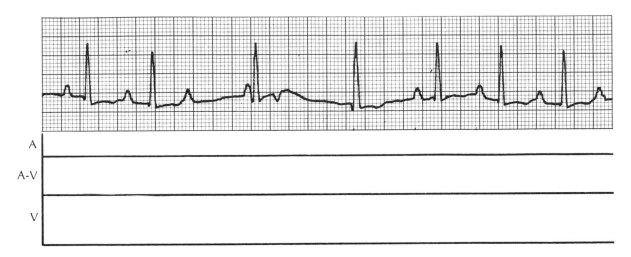

Conclusion: Your laddergram, properly done, will indicate that this is a type I second-degree heart block with two junctional escape beats. Compare your laddergram with the one below.

In place of the laddergram, the following explanation would be in order: The first two P waves are conducted with lengthening P-R intervals. The third P wave is not conducted, and before the fourth P wave has a chance to conduct, there is a junctional escape beat with retrograde atrial conduction. The next complex represents a junctional escape mechanism with simultaneous antegrade and retrograde conduction. After this, the sinus node resumes its role as pacemaker, and impulses are once again conducted with increasing P-R intervals. This is an atypical Wenckebach in that the second P-R interval does not have the greatest increment nor is there a shortening of the R-R interval.

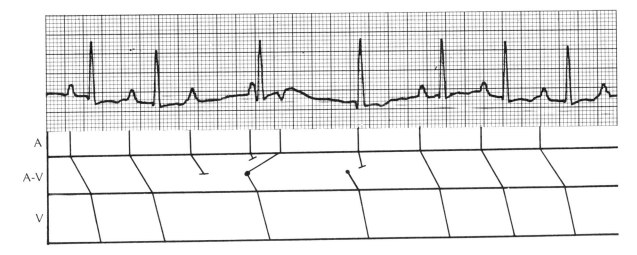

EXERCISE 6-9

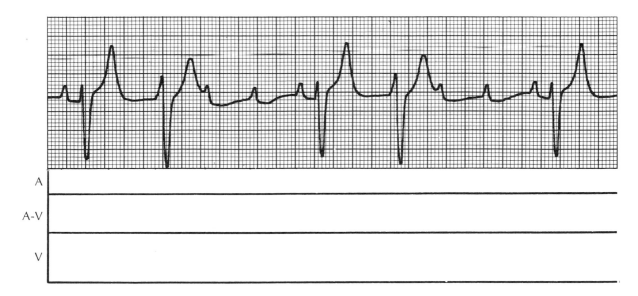

Conclusion: Here is one case in which a laddergram is necessary in order to establish the sequence of A-V conduction. As you mark off the P waves in the A tier, you are reminded that the sinus node is expected to beat at regular intervals. Thus you find P waves hidden in Ts and r waves. When it is time to draw the lines in the A-V tier, you note that the second beat of the pairs is not really as aberrant as it looks, since a P wave distorts it. It is a supraventricular beat conducted from the P in the preceding T—a Wenckebach (5:2) conduction pattern. There is an underlying sinus tachycardia.

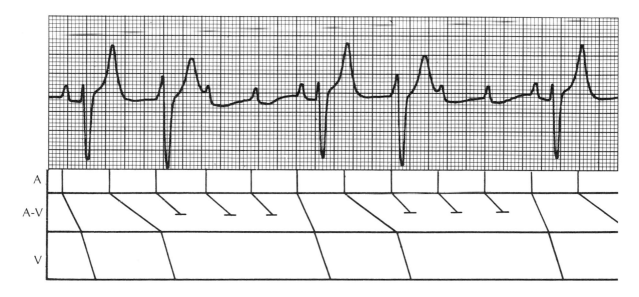

EXERCISE 6-10

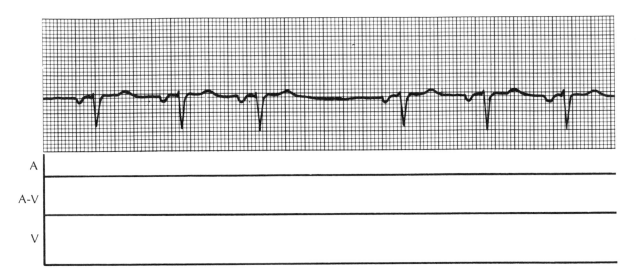

Conclusion: Aside from a lengthy explanation, a laddergram is probably the only clear way to illustrate the mechanism of this arrhythmia, although if you know the rules, you can easily diagnose it without a laddergram. The rules are: Shortening P-P intervals and a pause that is less than twice the shortest cycle indicate a Wenckebach mechanism. This is a sinus node Wenckebach.

In order to build the laddergrams, count the number of cycles in a group, including the dropped beat (a missing P in this case). Now divide this number (4) into the total length of the Wenckebach cycle (320 msec.), and you will come up with the interval between the firing of each sinus node beat (80 msec.). Start with the first P wave of a group and estimate a small amount of time for the sinus impulse to reach the atria. From this point walk out on the laddergram the sinus rhythm at the intervals you have calculated. This requires an additional tier at the top for S-A activity. Simply use the ECG graph. Draw in the P waves in the A tier. Draw a line from the point of sinus firing to the atrial line. The conduction time will be seen to increase each time until a beat is not conducted at all.

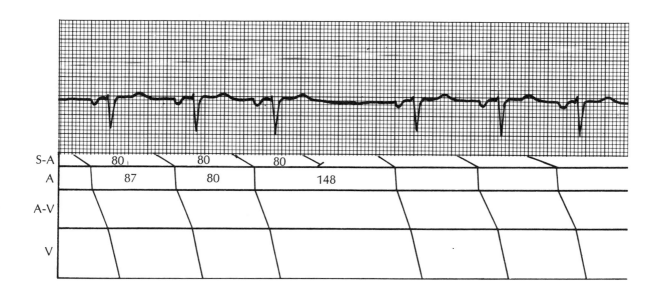

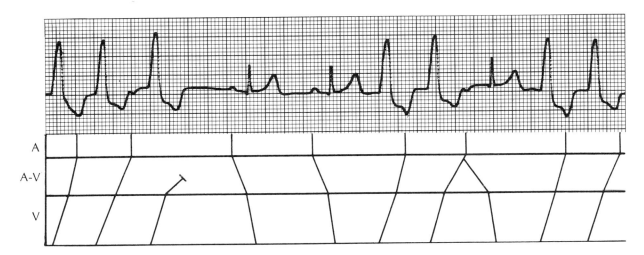

Conclusion: This is an interesting arrhythmia that might be missed without a laddergram. The first clue comes when you begin to mark off the P waves in the A tier. There are P waves after each PVC. The laddergram helps you to note that they are out of step with the sinus rhythm and therefore are retrograde P′ waves. Retrograde conduction time is seen to lengthen, and in the third PVC on the tracing retrograde conduction is blocked completely (a retrograde Wenckebach). The next time it happens there is a reciprocal beat; that is, the second retrograde P′ in the next set of PVCs travels back down the A-V junction to recapture the ventricles.

EXERCISE 6-12

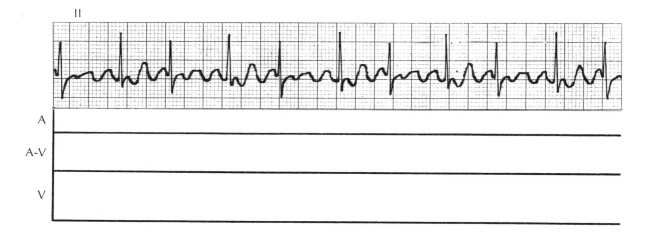

Conclusion: You will recognize the sawtooth pattern of atrial flutter quite readily in this tracing. The bigeminal rhythm, however, represents a more complicated mechanism. There is a Wenckebach mechanism in action. This is often the explanation when there is atrial flutter with alternating A-V conduction. Here we have a basic 2:1 block with the dropped beat every other cycle.

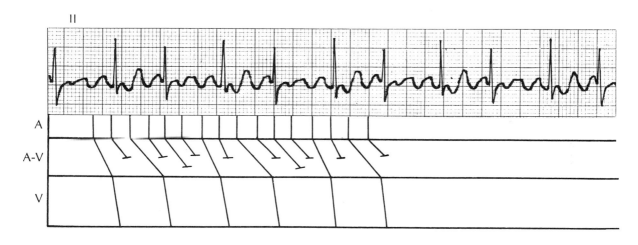

CHAPTER 7

HEMIBLOCK AND BUNDLE BRANCH BLOCK

In order to become proficient in the diagnosis of bundle branch block (BBB) and hemiblock, it is necessary to understand the lead systems, normal ECG, anatomy and physiology of the conductive system, coronary circulation, and mechanism of axis deviation. The following exercises will give you practice in the recognition of right bundle branch block (RBBB), left bundle branch block (LBBB), left anterior hemiblock (LAH), left posterior hemiblock (LPH), and the combinations of RBBB and hemiblock. Below are the ECG criteria for these conditions. If you find that your conclusions are wrong in the exercises, please refer back to these criteria.

RBBB

The only abnormality in uncomplicated RBBB is late activation of the right ventricle, which will be reflected by a broad QRS and by a late intrinsicoid deflection in lead V_1 (distance from onset of QRS to the peak of the R wave). Normally, in this lead, the R wave peaks at 0.02 sec. In RBBB the last R wave peaks at 0.06 sec. or more, and the QRS is usually triphasic. This late rightward activation will also produce a wide S wave in leads V_6 and I. In uncomplicated RBBB normal septal activation will be reflected by small q waves in leads I and V_6.

LBBB

In LBBB initial forces (septal) are abnormal (from right to left), and left ventricular activation is also abnormal and late. In uncomplicated LBBB the abnormal septal activation will be reflected by the absence of the normal little q waves in leads V_6 and I. Late activation of the left ventricle will be reflected by a broad QRS with a late intrinsicoid deflection in lead V_6. Lead I will have a monophasic R wave. Lead V_1 will be primarily negative. Sometimes lead V_1 will have a small, narrow r wave. This does not reflect normal septal activation. It simply implies that the anterior wall of the right ventricle was the first to activate.

LAH

The only ECG abnormality in uncomplicated LAH is left axis deviation (LAD) with a small r wave in the inferior leads (II, III, and aV_F) and a small q wave in lead I, reflecting septal activation, which is slightly inferior and from left to right. Axis deviation is determined in the frontal plane leads. When it is to the left, lead I will be positive, and leads II, III, and aV_F will be negative. Inferior wall myocardial infarction also has LAD; however, in this case the complex in the inferior leads will be a QS rather than an rS. When both inferior wall myocardial infarction and LAH are present, the hemiblock may mask the infarct by producing the little r in leads II, III, and aV_F.

LPH

The only ECG abnormality in uncomplicated LPH is right axis deviation (RAD). Again, the axis is determined in the frontal plane leads and cannot be seen in the precordial leads. RAD is +120° or more. In lead I the complex will be primarily negative (rS). Leads II and III will be primarily positive (qR). Note that RAD will be picked up only in lead I since the other two leads can be normally positive.

When a diagnosis of LPH is made, right ventricular hypertrophy must be ruled out since this condition will produce exactly the same pattern in the limb leads (RAD).

DETERMINING ELECTRICAL AXIS

As long as there is an equiphasic deflection in any one of the frontal plane leads, the axis can be determined in two easy steps. First, note that the equiphasic deflection indicates that the mean current is flowing perpendicular to the axis of that particular lead. Second, look at the lead whose axis is parallel to this current. The complex in that lead will be positive if the mean current is flowing toward the positive terminal and will be negative if it flows toward the negative terminal. For example, if the equiphasic deflection is in lead aV_R, you would determine if the axis is to the right or to the left by looking at lead III; and if the equiphasic deflection is in aV_F, you would make this determination by looking at lead I.

If there is not an equiphasic deflection in the six limb leads, there will be a third step. Choose the lead in which the complex is closest to equiphasic. Begin as though it is actually an equiphasic complex, remembering whether it is more negative or more positive. Proceed as in the first two steps. Now (third step), correct the

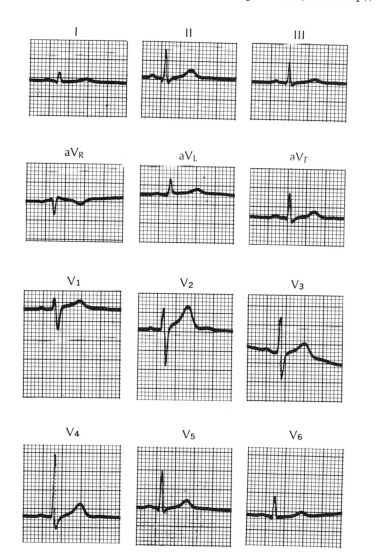

axis by tipping it slightly toward the positive of the equiphasic lead if the complex is more positive or slightly toward the negative if the complex is more negative.

NORMAL TWELVE-LEAD ECG

In the twelve-lead ECG displayed above, notice that the normal axis is reflected by a positive deflection in leads I, II, III, and aV_F. Leads III and aV_F can normally be negative, and lead II can be equiphasic and still present the picture of a normal axis.

Normal septal activation can be seen in leads I and V_6 (a little q wave). The QRS is of normal duration, as are the P-R and Q-T intervals. The R wave in the precordial leads gets larger, and the S waves get smaller from leads V_1 to V_4 (R wave progression).

EXERCISE 7-1

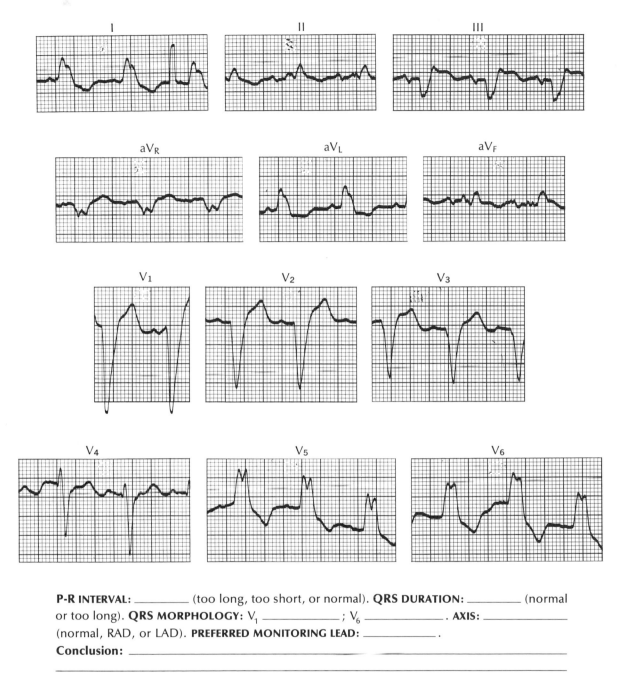

P-R INTERVAL: _____ (too long, too short, or normal). **QRS DURATION:** _____ (normal or too long). **QRS MORPHOLOGY:** V_1 _____ ; V_6 _____ . **AXIS:** _____ (normal, RAD, or LAD). **PREFERRED MONITORING LEAD:** _____ .
Conclusion: _____

_____

ANALYSIS

P-R INTERVAL: 0.16 sec. (normal). **QRS DURATION:** 0.20 sec. (too long). **QRS MORPHOLOGY:** V_1: QS; V_6: notched R. **AXIS:** normal. **PREFERRED MONITORING LEAD:** V_1 or MCL_1.
Conclusion: Certainly the most notable features of this electrocardiogram are the broad, slurred ventricular complexes that are completely negative in lead V_1. In LBBB the initial forces are altered, and ventricular depolarization commences in the septum from right to left. This is reflected in lead V_6 by absent q waves. Leads I and aV_L have a similar pattern because the positive terminals of these leads are on the left shoulder.

In uncomplicated LBBB the T wave polarity will be opposite the terminal part of the QRS.

You should have been able to determine the electrical axis of the heart by noting that the ventricular complex is almost isoelectric in lead aV_F (just slightly positive in value). Since lead I has an axis that is perpendicular to the axis of aV_F, you can now almost exactly determine the heart axis by the ventricular complex in this lead. It is totally positive. Therefore the main current flow of the heart is to the left, or toward the positive terminal of lead I and is almost perpendicular to aV_F but tipped a little toward the positive terminal. The electrical axis is approximately $+25°$. This is a normal axis, a common finding with LBBB.

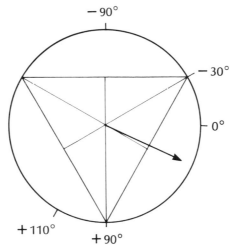

An electrical axis of $+25°$ would be perpendicular to the axis of aV_F and flowing into the positive terminal of lead I.

Your choice of a monitoring lead should depend on where the P wave is seen best.

EXERCISE 7-2

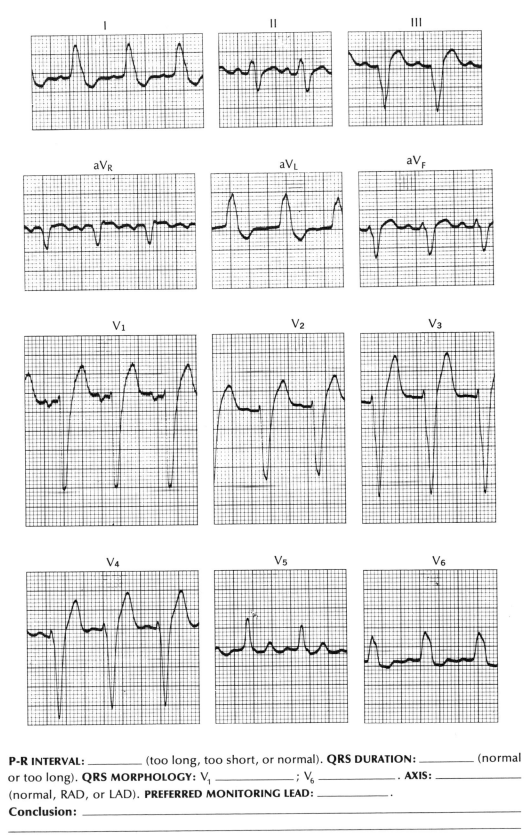

P-R INTERVAL: _____ (too long, too short, or normal). **QRS DURATION:** _____ (normal or too long). **QRS MORPHOLOGY:** V$_1$ _____ ; V$_6$ _____ . **AXIS:** _____ (normal, RAD, or LAD). **PREFERRED MONITORING LEAD:** _____ .

Conclusion: _____

_____

P-R INTERVAL: 0.16 sec. (normal). **QRS DURATION:** 0.14 sec. (too long). **QRS MORPHOLOGY:** V_1: rS; V_6: R. **AXIS:** normal. **PREFERRED MONITORING LEAD:** II.

Conclusion: The broad ventricular complexes, negative in V_1 are indicative of LBBB. The absence of normal septal activation is reflected by absent q waves in leads I, aV_L, and V_6. This patient should be monitored on the lead in which first-degree heart block will most easily be detected. In this case the P waves are seen best in lead II.

The electrical axis is determined by observing the equiphasic deflection in lead II and the fully positive value of aV_L, reflective of a current flowing perpendicular to the axis of lead II and full into the positive terminal of aV_L. The electrical axis of the heart is approximately $-30°$ (normal).

Note the small r wave in the right chest leads, indicating that initial activation took place in the anterior wall of the right ventricle.

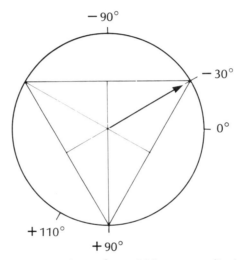

An electrical axis of $-30°$ would be perpendicular to the axis of lead II and flowing into the positive electrode of aV_L.

EXERCISE 7-3

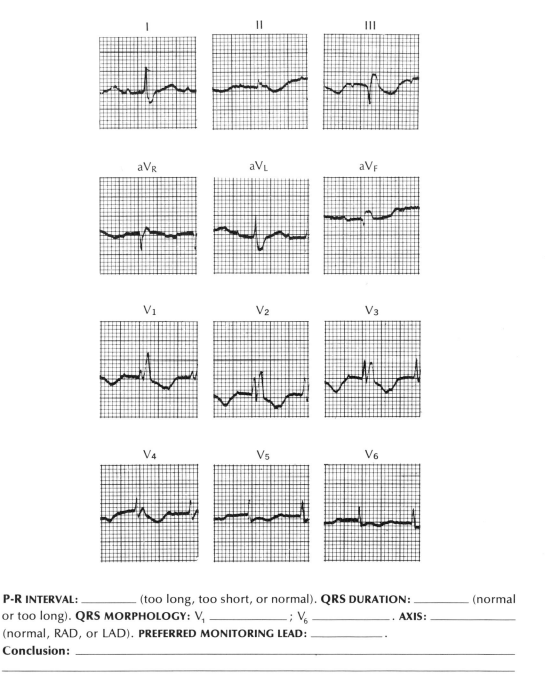

P-R INTERVAL: _____ (too long, too short, or normal). **QRS DURATION:** _____ (normal or too long). **QRS MORPHOLOGY:** V_1 _____ ; V_6 _____ . **AXIS:** _____ (normal, RAD, or LAD). **PREFERRED MONITORING LEAD:** _____ .

Conclusion: _____

_____

ANALYSIS

P-R INTERVAL: 0.16 sec. (normal). **QRS DURATION:** 0.12 sec. (too long). **QRS MORPHOLOGY:** V_1: rsR′; V_6: Rs. **AXIS:** normal. **PREFERRED MONITORING LEAD:** II and occasional checks on I.

Conclusion: Notice the predominantly positive deflection (M shaped) in lead V_1. Remember that the ventricular complex in this lead is usually an rS configuration, with the small initial r wave reflecting septal depolarization and the deep S wave reflecting left ventricular depolarization. In RBBB the initial forces and left ventricular activation are normal. In lead V_1 this would be reflected in a small r and an S wave. However, since the right ventricle is depolarized late, this deflection would no longer be lost in the left ventricular complex but would be quite visible as a late strong positive terminal event (R'). Leads I and V₆ would also reflect this late activation of the right ventricle in a broad S wave, indicating late terminal vector forces directed to the right (away from leads I and V₆).

Here again the electrical axis can be estimated simply by observing the six limb leads for an equiphasic deflection. This is found in aV$_F$ and indicates that the main direction of current flow is perpendicular, or almost perpendicular, to the axis of this lead. Knowing the main direction of current flow, however, does not tell you whether the current flows to the right or to the left. The lead whose axis is perpendicular to that of aV$_F$ is lead I. Note that the ventricular complex is primarily positive in this lead, indicating that the main current flow is to the left. Since the aV$_F$ complex was not exactly equiphasic (slightly more positive than negative), we can now make a small correction toward the positive terminal of aV$_F$. The estimated axis is +10°.

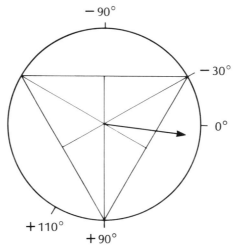

An electrical axis of +10° would be perpendicular to the axis of aV$_F$ and flowing into the positive terminal of lead I.

Any patient with RBBB should be monitored mainly on lead II with occasional checks on lead I. The reason for this is that since you already know that the right bundle is blocked, monitoring on lead V₁ will give you no new information. If one of the left fascicles also becomes blocked, you would pick this up on lead II (LAH) or lead I (LPH).

EXERCISE 7-4

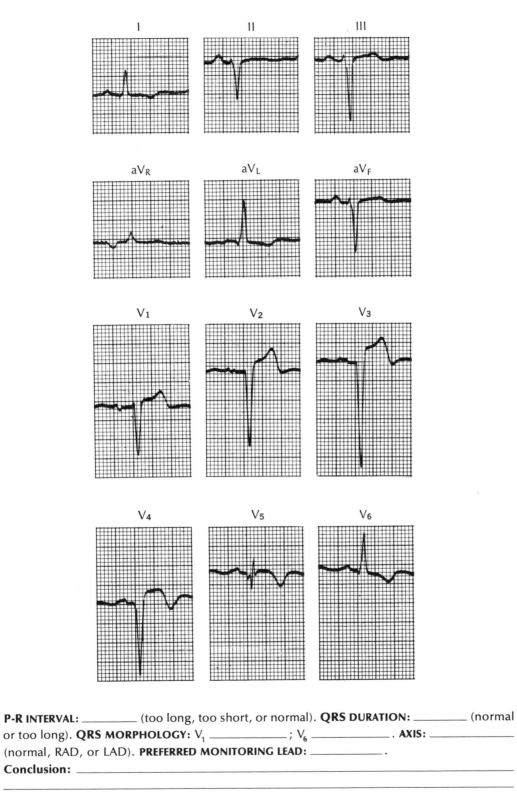

P-R INTERVAL: _____ (too long, too short, or normal). **QRS DURATION:** _____ (normal or too long). **QRS MORPHOLOGY:** V_1 _____ ; V_6 _____ . **AXIS:** _____ (normal, RAD, or LAD). **PREFERRED MONITORING LEAD:** _____ .

Conclusion: _____

_____

ANALYSIS

P-R INTERVAL: 0.16 sec. (normal). **QRS DURATION:** 0.10 sec. (normal). **QRS MORPHOLOGY:** V_1: QS; V_6: qR. **AXIS:** LAD. **PREFERRED MONITORING LEAD:** V_1 or MCL_1.

Conclusion: Immediately apparent in this twelve-lead ECG is the abnormal left axis deviation (LAD), as reflected by the deep negative complexes in leads II, III, and aV$_F$. This rS pattern, along with the qR pattern in lead I, is diagnostic of LAH. A glance at lead V$_1$ indicates that the right bundle branch is still intact. Since you already know that this patient has LAH, monitoring him on lead II would run the risk of missing a developing RBBB. You would therefore choose V$_1$ or MCL$_1$ as a monitoring lead, with occasional checks on lead II to see if the hemiblock pattern still persists. You will notice that the R wave progression in the precordial leads is lost. This may indicate an anteroseptal myocardial infarction, which is discussed in Chapter 9.

To determine the electrical axis by estimation, you would find an equiphasic deflection in one of the limb leads. Lead aV$_R$ is not equiphasic, but it is the smallest deflection, indicating that the main current flow crosses the axis of this lead almost on a perpendicular. Now, the axis of lead III is also perpendicular to the axis of this lead. The strong negative deflection in lead III indicates that the main current flow is toward the negative terminal of that lead, which places the electrical axis at approximately −60°.

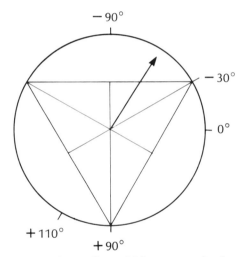

An electrical axis of − 60° would be perpendicular to the axis of aV$_R$ and flowing into the negative terminal of lead III.

EXERCISE 7-5

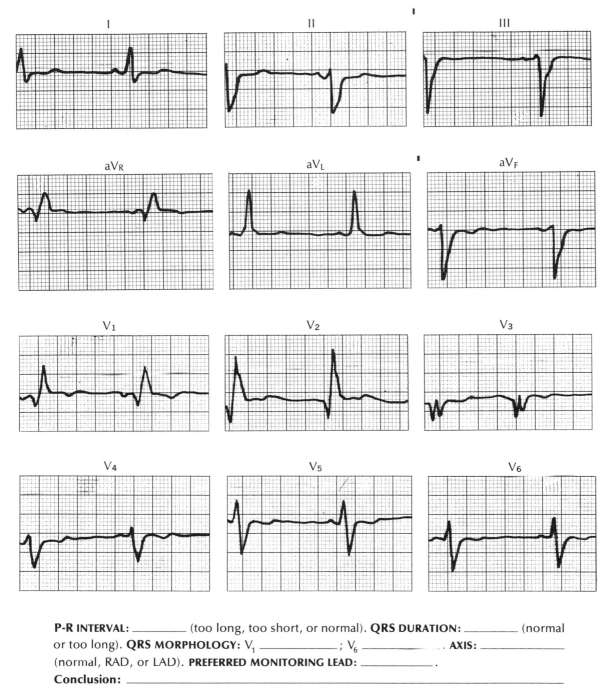

P-R INTERVAL: _____ (too long, too short, or normal). **QRS DURATION:** _____ (normal or too long). **QRS MORPHOLOGY:** V_1 _____ ; V_6 _____ . **AXIS:** _____ (normal, RAD, or LAD). **PREFERRED MONITORING LEAD:** _____ .
Conclusion: _____

ANALYSIS

P-R INTERVAL: 0.14 sec. (normal). **QRS DURATION:** 0.18 sec. (too long). **QRS MORPHOLOGY:** V_1: qR; V_6: RS. **AXIS:** LAD. **PREFERRED MONITORING LEAD:** I, V_1, or MCL$_1$.
Conclusion: The broad terminal R wave in lead V_1 indicates late activation of the right ventricle, and the rS pattern in leads II, III, and aV$_F$ indicates abnormal LAD. The diagnosis is, then, RBBB and LAH (bifascicular block). This patient should be monitored on the lead in which the P waves can be seen best, since the appearance of a first-degree heart block would indicate that the remaining fascicle (the posterior

division of the left bundle) may be also blocked. When all three fascicles are involved, the term trifascicular block is used.

Here again, the electrical axis is estimated by looking at the six limb leads for an equiphasic, or nearly equiphasic, deflection. This is found in lead aV_R, where the complex is more positive than it is negative but is the closest to being isoelectric. You can therefore surmise that the main current flow is almost perpendicular to the axis of aV_R. However, you do not know whether the current goes to the left or the right. Since the axis of lead III is also perpendicular to the axis of aV_R, you have a good guide for determining the direction. Lead III is strongly negative, indicating that the current flows toward the negative terminal of this lead and thus that the axis of the heart is mainly to the left. To be more specific, you can now take into account the more positive value of aV_R and swing the axis a little more toward that lead's positive electrode, which would bring the electrical axis of the heart somewhere between −60° and −65°.

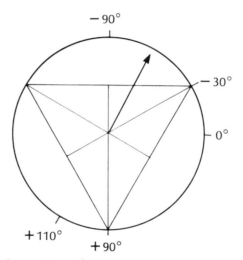

An electrical axis of −65° would be almost perpendicular to the axis of aV_R and flowing toward the negative terminal of lead III.

EXERCISE 7-6

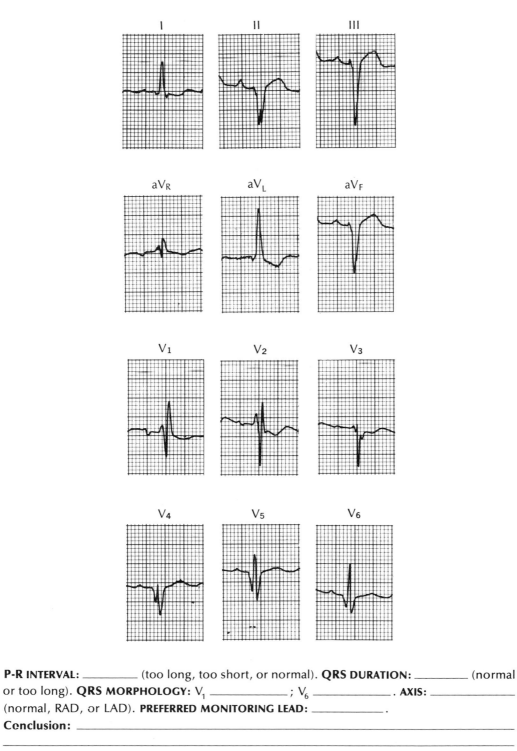

P-R INTERVAL: _____ (too long, too short, or normal). **QRS DURATION:** _____ (normal or too long). **QRS MORPHOLOGY:** V_1 _____; V_6 _____. **AXIS:** _____ (normal, RAD, or LAD). **PREFERRED MONITORING LEAD:** _____ .

Conclusion: _____

_____

ANALYSIS

P-R INTERVAL: 0.16 sec. (normal). **QRS DURATION:** 0.12 sec. (too long). **QRS MORPHOLOGY:** V_1: rSR′; V_6: qRs. **AXIS:** LAD. **PREFERRED MONITORING LEAD:** II.

Conclusion: In lead V_1 of this ECG it is possible to see the deflections resulting from depolarization of both the left and the right ventricles. The small initial r wave represents normal septal depolarization from left to right, or toward the positive terminal of this lead. The deep S wave reflects normal left ventricular depolarization, and the terminal R' wave is a telltale sign of late activation of the right ventricle (RBBB). Ordinarily, the right ventricular force is lost in the greater force of the left ventricle when both ventricles depolarize together as they should. This delayed right ventricular activation can also be seen in the left precordial leads and in lead I as a broad terminal S wave, reflective of a force traveling away from these positive terminals.

The electrical axis of this patient's heart is best determined from leads aV$_R$ and III. It is almost perpendicular to the axis of aV$_R$ and directed toward the negative terminal of III, placing the main current flow toward the left shoulder. This, combined with the qR in I and the rS in II and aV$_F$, is diagnostic of LAH. The patient has two out of the three known ventricular bundle branches blocked. He should therefore be monitored very closely for a lengthening P-R interval, which would indicate the development of further block. The P wave in this patient is best seen in lead II, which should be your monitoring lead.

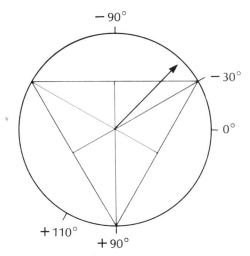

An electrical axis of −45° would be perpendicular to the axis of aV$_R$ and flowing into the positive terminal of lead III.

EXERCISE 7-7

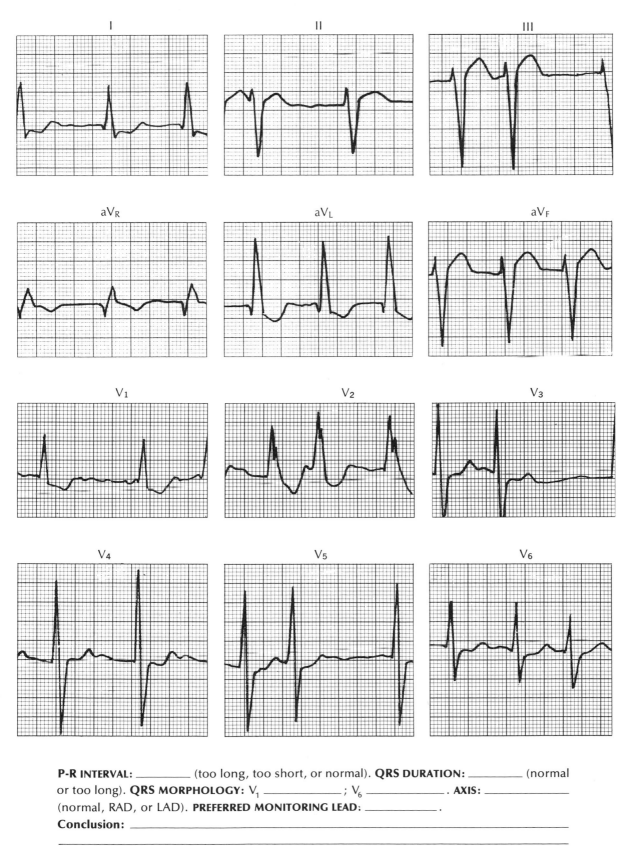

P-R INTERVAL: _____ (too long, too short, or normal). **QRS DURATION:** _____ (normal or too long). **QRS MORPHOLOGY:** V_1 _____ ; V_6 _____ . **AXIS:** _____ (normal, RAD, or LAD). **PREFERRED MONITORING LEAD:** _____ .

Conclusion: _____

_____

P-R INTERVAL: absent P waves. **QRS DURATION:** 0.16 sec. (too long). **QRS MORPHOLOGY:** V_1: qR; V_6: qRS. **AXIS:** LAD. **PREFERRED MONITORING LEADS:** II and V_1 or MCL_1.

Conclusion: The broad terminal R wave in lead V_1 is abnormal and indicates a late current flowing toward the electrode of this lead, which is a sign of late activation of the right ventricle (RBBB). Since you know that the right bundle and the anterior division of the left bundle have a common anatomical origin and a common blood supply (anterior descending branch of the left coronary artery), you will be on the alert for a coexisting block of the left anterior fascicle. This is clearly evident in the left axis deviation, reflected by the rS complexes seen in leads II, III, and aV_F, and the qRs of lead I of this patient. There is, then, a block of two of the three known fascicles of the ventricular conductive system. Ordinarily, at this point you would be concerned about the prolongation of the P-R interval, indicating involvement of the only remaining fascicle. However, this patient has atrial fibrillation, and recognition of involvement of the posterior fascicle by a very slow idioventricular rhythm (trifascicular block) would probably come too late.

Estimation of the electrical axis is easily made by observing the almost equiphasic complex in aV_R and the negative complex in III. These complexes indicate that the mean electrical axis is directed up toward the left shoulder, with slightly more value toward the positive pole of aV_R—at about $-60°$.

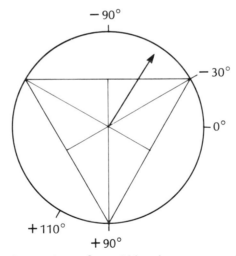

An electrical axis of $-60°$ would be almost perpendicular to the axis of aV_R and flowing more toward the negative terminal of lead III.

EXERCISE 7-8

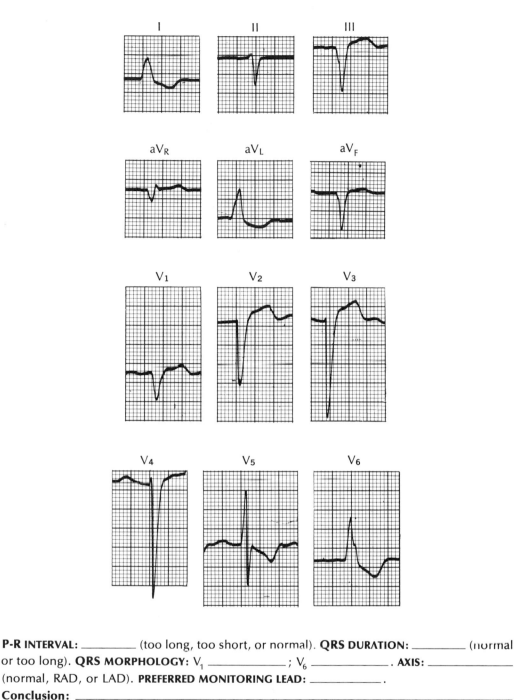

P-R INTERVAL: _____ (too long, too short, or normal). **QRS DURATION:** _____ (normal or too long). **QRS MORPHOLOGY:** V$_1$ _____ ; V$_6$ _____ . **AXIS:** _____ (normal, RAD, or LAD). **PREFERRED MONITORING LEAD:** _____ .
Conclusion: _____

ANALYSIS

P-R INTERVAL: absent P waves. **QRS DURATION:** 0.14 sec. (too long). **QRS MORPHOLOGY:** V$_1$: QS; V$_6$: R. **AXIS:** LAD. **PREFERRED MONITORING LEAD:** immaterial.
Conclusion: This is LBBB with LAD. P waves are not seen because of atrial fibrillation. The axis does not always shift to the left with LBBB. When it does, it is thought to indicate an incomplete BBB with a complete LAH.

Note the absence of Q waves in I, aV$_L$ and V$_6$, which is reflective of abnormal septal activation.

EXERCISE 7-9

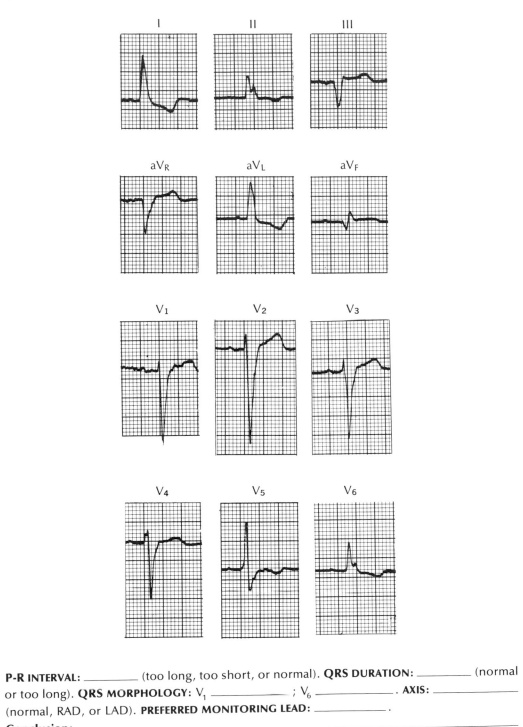

P-R INTERVAL: _____ (too long, too short, or normal). **QRS DURATION:** _____ (normal or too long). **QRS MORPHOLOGY:** V₁ _____ ; V₆ _____ . **AXIS:** _____ (normal, RAD, or LAD). **PREFERRED MONITORING LEAD:** _____ .

Conclusion: _____

ANALYSIS

P-R INTERVAL: 0.17 sec. (normal). **QRS DURATION:** 0.14 sec. (too long). **QRS MORPHOLOGY:** V_1: rS; V_6: R. **AXIS:** normal. **PREFERRED MONITORING LEAD:** V_1.

Conclusion: This is LBBB. Note the narrow r wave in lead V_1. This occurs about 30% of the time in LBBB and is probably reflective of initial activation of the anterior right ventricular wall.[3] The presence of this small narrow r wave in LBBB aberration helps one to distinguish between it and right ventricular ectopy.

EXERCISE 7-10

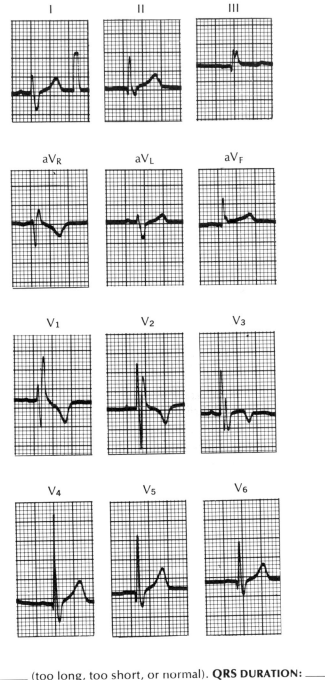

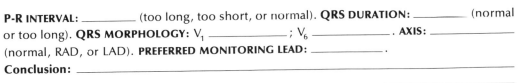

P-R INTERVAL: _____ (too long, too short, or normal). **QRS DURATION:** _____ (normal or too long). **QRS MORPHOLOGY:** V_1 _____ ; V_6 _____ . **AXIS:** _____ (normal, RAD, or LAD). **PREFERRED MONITORING LEAD:** _____ .

Conclusion: _____

_____

ANALYSIS

P-R INTERVAL: 0.14 sec. (normal). **QRS DURATION:** 0.12 sec. (too long). **QRS MORPHOLOGY:** V_1: rSR′; V_6: qRs. **AXIS:** normal. **PREFERRED MONITORING LEAD:** II with checks on I. **Conclusion:** This is RBBB with a normal axis. The patient should be monitored on lead II to watch for the development of LAD, which is reflective of LAH. It is also possible that LPH could ensue. Therefore an occasional check on lead I is necessary. RAD will cause *lead I* to become almost completely negative (rS), and LAD will cause *lead II* to become almost completely negative (rS).

EXERCISE 7-11

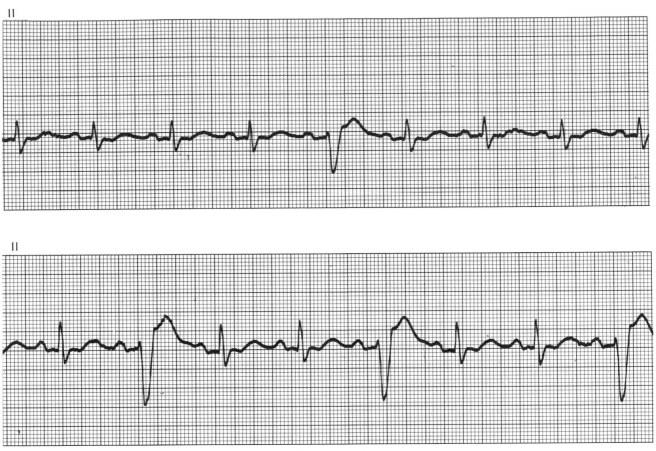

Same patient.

RATE: _____ (normal, bradycardia, or tachycardia). **RHYTHM:** _____ (regular or irregular) _____ (ventricular or supraventricular). **P-R INTERVAL:** _____ (too long, too short, or normal) _____ (absent P waves). **QRS DURATION:** _____ (normal or too long). **Q-T INTERVAL:** _____ (normal, too long, or too short). **P' WAVES:** _____ (present or absent). **JUNCTIONAL ECTOPIC BEATS:** _____ (present or absent). **VENTRICULAR ECTOPIC BEATS:** _____ (present or absent) _____ (unifocal or multifocal) _____ (frequent or infrequent) _____ (R on T).

Conclusion: _____

_____

ANALYSIS

RATE: 73/min. (normal). **RHYTHM:** regular and supraventricular. **P-R INTERVAL:** 0.24 sec. (too long). **QRS DURATION:** 0.13 sec. (too long). **Q-T INTERVAL:** 0.50 sec. (too long). **P' WAVES:** absent. **JUNCTIONAL ECTOPIC BEATS:** absent. **VENTRICULAR ECTOPIC BEATS:** absent. **Conclusion:** This patient has intermittent LAH, which began with an occasional block and then occurred every third beat. There is also first-degree heart block. The twelve-lead ECG displayed below is from the same patient later and indicates that the broad QRS seen in the above tracings is reflective of RBBB.

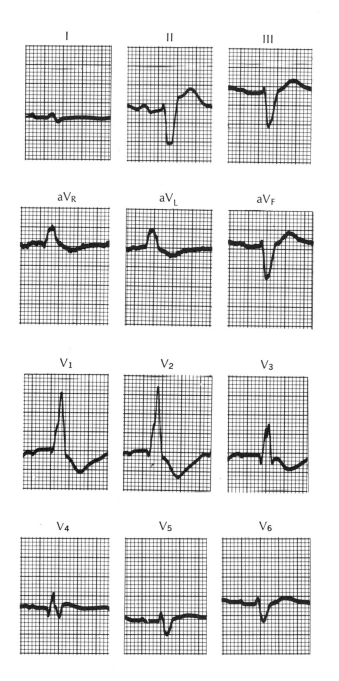

This is an example of trifascicular block—RBBB, LAH, and first-degree heart block. It is called trifascicular because two fascicles are obviously blocked, and the third (posterior division of the left bundle) probably has a partial block, reflected by the prolonged P-R interval. The first-degree heart block could, of course, be in the bundle of His or above. However, with two fascicles already blocked, it is safer to consider that any further block involves the only remaining fascicle. If LPH ensues, the idioventricular rhythm may be below 30/min.

EXERCISE 7-12

V₁

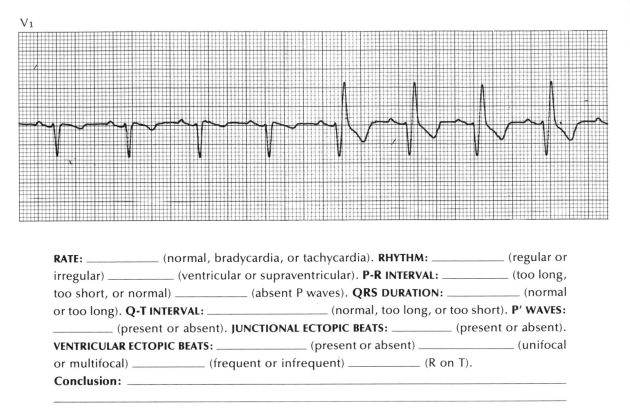

RATE: _____ (normal, bradycardia, or tachycardia). **RHYTHM:** _____ (regular or irregular) _____ (ventricular or supraventricular). **P-R INTERVAL:** _____ (too long, too short, or normal) _____ (absent P waves). **QRS DURATION:** _____ (normal or too long). **Q-T INTERVAL:** _____ (normal, too long, or too short). **P' WAVES:** _____ (present or absent). **JUNCTIONAL ECTOPIC BEATS:** _____ (present or absent). **VENTRICULAR ECTOPIC BEATS:** _____ (present or absent) _____ (unifocal or multifocal) _____ (frequent or infrequent) _____ (R on T). **Conclusion:** _____

ANALYSIS

RATE: 82/min. (normal). **RHYTHM:** regular and supraventricular. **P-R INTERVAL:** 0.11 sec. (normal). **QRS DURATION:** 0.09 and 0.15 sec. (normal and too long). **Q-T INTERVAL:** 0.34 sec. (normal). **P' WAVES:** absent. **JUNCTIONAL ECTOPIC BEATS:** absent. **VENTRICULAR ECTOPIC BEATS:** absent.

Conclusion: Here you see the sudden onset of RBBB. You may have been inclined to call this ventricular ectopy. However, the broad beats are not premature since the P-R interval does not change. They have the classical morphology of RBBB, as seen in V₁ (rSR'). The only change in the complex is the appearance of a late R' wave, reflective of late activation of the right ventricle.

EXERCISE 7-13

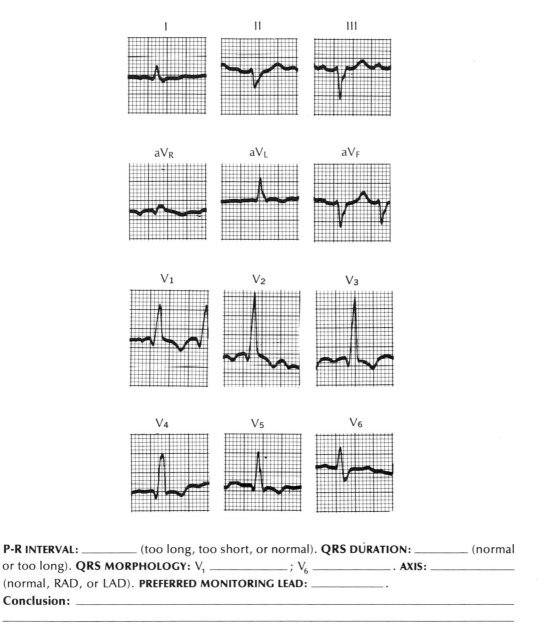

P-R INTERVAL: _____ (too long, too short, or normal). **QRS DURATION:** _____ (normal or too long). **QRS MORPHOLOGY:** V$_1$ _____ ; V$_6$ _____ . **AXIS:** _____ (normal, RAD, or LAD). **PREFERRED MONITORING LEAD:** _____ .

Conclusion: _____

_____

ANALYSIS

P-R INTERVAL: 0.18 sec. (normal). **QRS DURATION:** 0.13 sec. (too long). **QRS MORPHOLOGY:** V$_1$: qR; V$_6$: RS. **AXIS:** LAD. **PREFERRED MONITORING LEAD:** III.

Conclusion: This is a bifascicular block—RBBB and LAH. You will monitor on the lead in which the P waves are best seen. Note the abnormal q waves and T-wave inversion in the chest leads from V$_1$ to V$_5$ and the absence of normal q waves in leads I and V$_6$. This is an anterior septal myocardial infarction and is discussed in Chapter 8 on myocardial infarction.

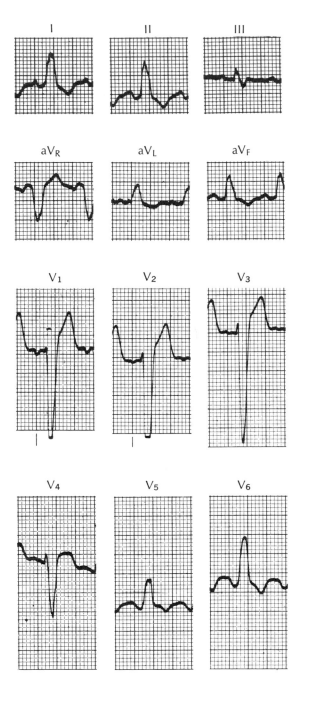

P-R INTERVAL: _____ (too long, too short, or normal). **QRS DURATION:** _____ (normal or too long). **QRS MORPHOLOGY:** V₁ _____ ; V₆ _____ . **AXIS:** _____ (normal, RAD, or LAD). **PREFERRED MONITORING LEAD:** _____ .

Conclusion: _____

_____

ANALYSIS

P-R INTERVAL: 0.12 sec. (normal). **QRS DURATION:** 0.15 sec. (too long). **QRS MORPHOLOGY:** V₁: rS; V₆: R. **AXIS:** normal. **PREFERRED MONITORING LEAD:** immaterial.
Conclusion: LBBB.

EXERCISE 7-15

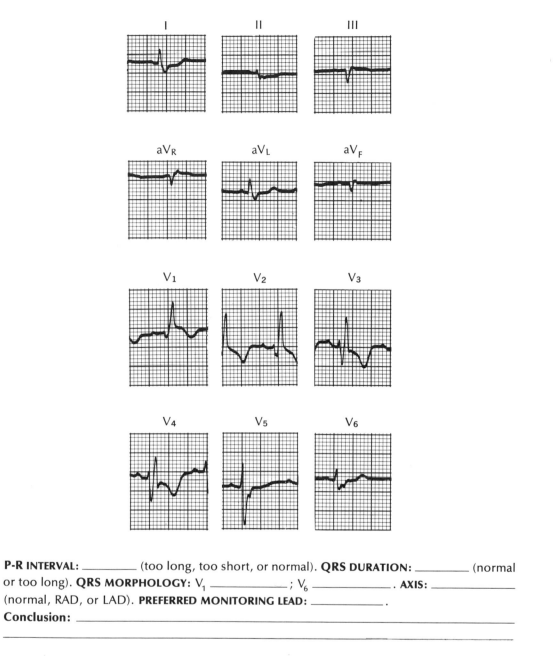

P-R INTERVAL: _____ (too long, too short, or normal). **QRS DURATION:** _____ (normal or too long). **QRS MORPHOLOGY:** V$_1$ _____ ; V$_6$ _____ . **AXIS:** _____ (normal, RAD, or LAD). **PREFERRED MONITORING LEAD:** _____ .
Conclusion: _____

ANALYSIS

P-R INTERVAL: 0.12 sec. (normal). **QRS DURATION:** 0.12 sec. (too long). **QRS MORPHOLOGY:** V$_1$: qR; V$_6$: RS. **AXIS:** normal. **PREFERRED MONITORING LEAD:** II with checks on I.
Conclusion: RBBB.

EXERCISE 7-16

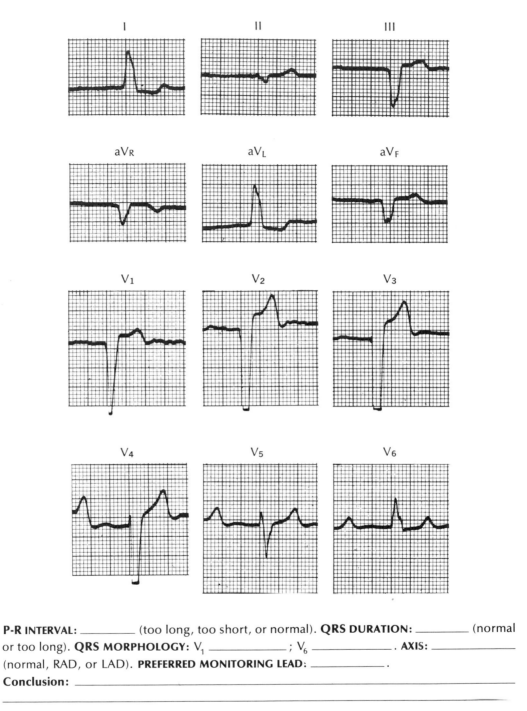

P-R INTERVAL: _____ (too long, too short, or normal). **QRS DURATION:** _____ (normal or too long). **QRS MORPHOLOGY:** V$_1$ _____ ; V$_6$ _____ . **AXIS:** _____ (normal, RAD, or LAD). **PREFERRED MONITORING LEAD:** _____ .
Conclusion: _____

ANALYSIS

P-R INTERVAL: absent P waves. **QRS DURATION:** 0.14 sec. (too long). **QRS MORPHOLOGY:** V$_1$: QS; V$_6$: R. **AXIS:** LAD. **PREFERRED MONITORING LEAD:** immaterial.
Conclusion: LBBB and atrial fibrillation.

EXERCISE 7-17

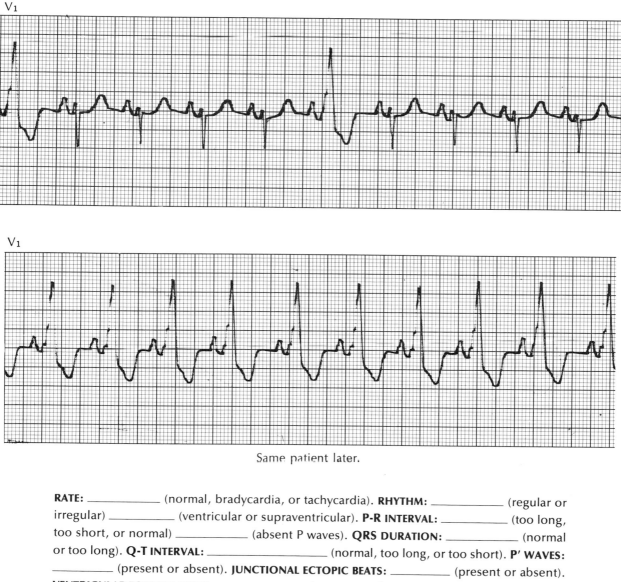

Same patient later.

RATE: _____ (normal, bradycardia, or tachycardia). **RHYTHM:** _____ (regular or irregular) _____ (ventricular or supraventricular). **P-R INTERVAL:** _____ (too long, too short, or normal) _____ (absent P waves). **QRS DURATION:** _____ (normal or too long). **Q-T INTERVAL:** _____ (normal, too long, or too short). **P' WAVES:** _____ (present or absent). **JUNCTIONAL ECTOPIC BEATS:** _____ (present or absent). **VENTRICULAR ECTOPIC BEATS:** _____ (present or absent) _____ (unifocal or multifocal) _____ (frequent or infrequent) _____ (R on T). **Conclusion:** _____ _____

_____

ANALYSIS

RATE: 90/min. (normal). **P-R INTERVAL:** 0.14 sec. (normal). **QRS DURATION:** 0.08 and 0.17 sec. (normal and too long). **Q-T INTERVAL:** 0.36 sec. (normal). **P' WAVES:** absent. **JUNCTIONAL ECTOPIC BEATS:** absent. **VENTRICULAR ECTOPIC BEATS:** absent.

Conclusion: The intermittent RBBB in the top tracing later becomes a sustained RBBB. In the top tracing the broad beats might have been mistaken for end diastolic PVCs. However the P-R interval does not change before the anomalous complexes. They are conducted beats.

EXERCISE 7-18

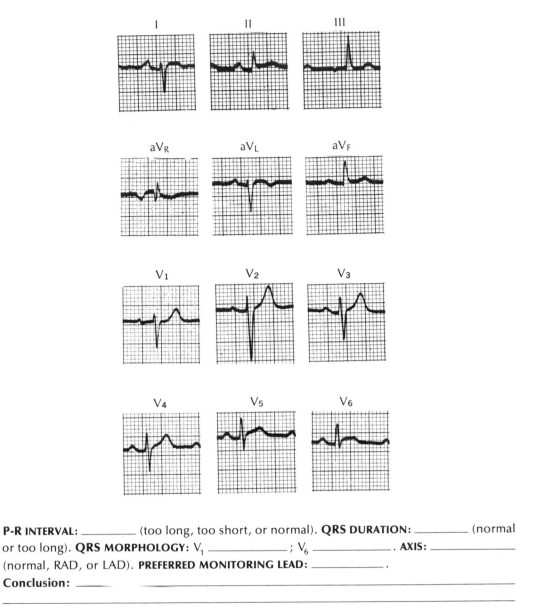

P-R INTERVAL: _____ (too long, too short, or normal). **QRS DURATION:** _____ (normal or too long). **QRS MORPHOLOGY:** V₁ _____ ; V₆ _____ . **AXIS:** _____ (normal, RAD, or LAD). **PREFERRED MONITORING LEAD:** _____ .
Conclusion: _____ _____

ANALYSIS

P-R INTERVAL: 0.16 sec. (normal). **QRS DURATION:** 0.08 sec. (normal). **QRS MORPHOLOGY:** V₁: rS; V₆: qRs. **AXIS:** RAD. **PREFERRED MONITORING LEAD:** V₁.
Conclusion: This is LPH.

CHAPTER 8

ABERRANT VENTRICULAR CONDUCTION

In this chapter you will be given exercises to help you to learn the different mechanisms involved in a ventricular ectopic beat, as opposed to aberrant ventricular conduction, and to know when you can and cannot tell the difference between the two.

Eighty percent of all aberrancies will be RBBB; the remainder will be LBBB and hemiblock. The frequency of RBBB aberrancy is due to the fact that the right bundle takes longer to repolarize than the left bundle. Therefore, a PAC occurring early enough is more likely to find the right bundle still repolarizing and unable to conduct, hence an RBBB pattern.

At times a supraventricular tachycardia with aberrant ventricular conduction will exactly simulate ventricular tachycardia, and a PAC with aberrancy will simulate a PVC. It is important to know how to tell the difference between the two and just as important to know when it is impossible to tell the difference with the surface ECG. Without using invasive methods, we have the following clues: (1) P waves, (2) morphology of the ventricular complex in leads V_1 and V_6, and (3) heart sounds and neck veins.

P WAVES

If you can see a premature P′ wave preceding the anomalous complex, then you usually need not be concerned with the morphology of the ventricular complex. The PAC is evident, and aberrant ventricular conduction is assumed. Most often the P′ wave will have to be detected, since if it is early enough to cause aberration, it will probably be hidden in the T wave. Just be sure that the P wave in question is actually premature and that you are not dealing with an end-diastolic PVC.

MORPHOLOGY

When you cannot see a P′ wave, you will be required to differentiate morphologically between left ventricular ectopy and RBBB aberration, since both are primarily positive in lead V_1. On fewer occasions it will be necessary to differentiate between right ventricular ectopy and LBBB aberration, since both are primarily negative in lead V_1. Sometimes there are no morphological clues.

The following approximate odds are given by Dr. H. J. L. Marriott.

RBBB aberrancy will sometimes manifest with the classical triphasic rSR′ pattern in V_1 and qRs in V_6. When it does, the odds are in favor of aberration; 10:1 in V_1 and 20:1 in V_6.

Left ventricular ectopy is also positive in V_1, but it is more likely to be monophasic or to have a qR. In addition, if there are two peaks, the first peak is more likely to be higher. (A higher second peak is useless as a clue.) With these occurrences, the odds are 10:1 in favor of ectopy. A QS in V_6 will give you 20:1 odds.

When differentiating between LBBB aberrancy and right ventricular ectopy, we do not have as many morphological clues. If there is an rS complex in lead V_1, the r wave may be fat in ectopy (broader than 0.03 sec.), whereas in LBBB it will almost always be narrow. This morphological clue offers 10:1 odds.

The following clinical clues are helpful in differentiating between aberrancy and ectopy. First, listen to the first heart sound while the patient holds his breath. It will be of varying intensity in ventricular tachycardia. Exceptions to this would be ventricular tachycardia with 1:1 retrograde conduction to the atria and ventricular tachycardia with atrial fibrillation.

In supraventricular tachycardia the first heart sound will be of unvarying intensity while the patient is holding his breath. An exception to this would be junctional tachycardia with A-V dissociation.

Second, look at the neck veins. Irregular cannon waves imply ventricular tachycardia. Regular cannon waves or none at all imply supraventricular tachycardia. The above exceptions will also apply.

Finally, carotid sinus pressure may terminate a supraventricular tachycardia.

EXERCISE 8-1

V$_1$

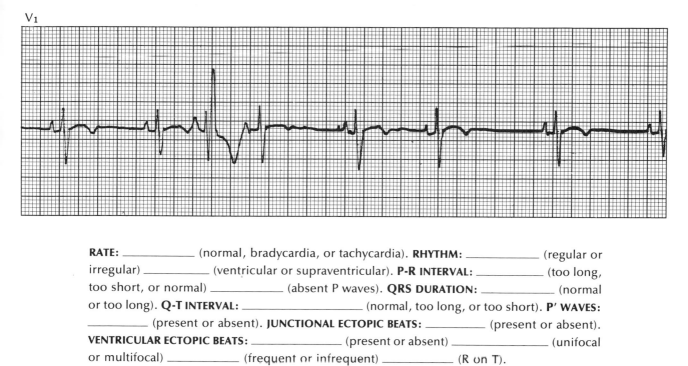

RATE: _____ (normal, bradycardia, or tachycardia). **RHYTHM:** _____ (regular or irregular) _____ (ventricular or supraventricular). **P-R INTERVAL:** _____ (too long, too short, or normal) _____ (absent P waves). **QRS DURATION:** _____ (normal or too long). **Q-T INTERVAL:** _____ (normal, too long, or too short). **P' WAVES:** _____ (present or absent). **JUNCTIONAL ECTOPIC BEATS:** _____ (present or absent). **VENTRICULAR ECTOPIC BEATS:** _____ (present or absent) _____ (unifocal or multifocal) _____ (frequent or infrequent) _____ (R on T). **Conclusion:** _____

_____

ANALYSIS

RATE: 50-100/min. (bradycardia). **RHYTHM:** irregular and supraventricular. **P-R INTERVAL:** 0.12 sec. (normal). **QRS DURATION:** 0.08 sec. (normal). **Q-T INTERVAL:** 0.37 sec. (too short). **P' WAVES:** present. **JUNCTIONAL ECTOPIC BEATS:** absent. **VENTRICULAR ECTOPIC BEATS:** absent.

Conclusion: The PAC before the anomalous-looking beat is easily seen. It is conducted with RBBB aberration. An atrial echo follows with a ventricular reciprocal beat. Another atrial echo is blocked, and the sinus rhythm recommences, only to be interrupted by another PAC. This time conduction is normal becaue the P' wave occurs later in the cycle.

EXERCISE 8-2

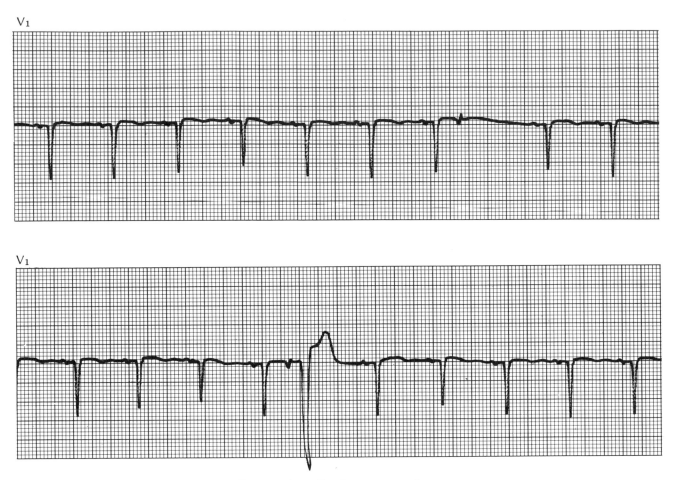

V₁

V₁

Same patient. Tracings not continuous.

RATE: _____ (normal, bradycardia, or tachycardia). **RHYTHM:** _____ (regular or irregular) _____ (ventricular or supraventricular). **P-R INTERVAL:** _____ (too long, too short, or normal) _____ (absent P waves). **QRS DURATION:** _____ (normal or too long). **Q-T INTERVAL:** _____ (normal, too long, or too short). **P′ WAVES:** _____ (present or absent). **JUNCTIONAL ECTOPIC BEATS:** _____ (present or absent). **VENTRICULAR ECTOPIC BEATS:** _____ (present or absent) _____ (unifocal or multifocal) _____ (frequent or infrequent) _____ (R on T). **Conclusion:** _____

ANALYSIS

RATE: 80-100/min. (normal). **RHYTHM:** irregular and supraventricular. **P-R INTERVAL:** 0.15 sec. (normal). **QRS DURATION:** 0.07 sec. (normal). **Q-T INTERVAL:** 0.36 sec. (normal). **P′ WAVES:** present. **JUNCTIONAL ECTOPIC BEATS:** absent. **VENTRICULAR ECTOPIC BEATS:** absent. **Conclusion:** There is a nonconducted PAC in the first tracing. In the second tracing the PAC is conducted with LBBB aberration.

If the P′ wave were not so evident, the less-than-full compensatory pause would have helped to indicate atrial ectopy. Morphologically there would be no clues since an initial r wave is not present.

EXERCISE 8-3

V₁

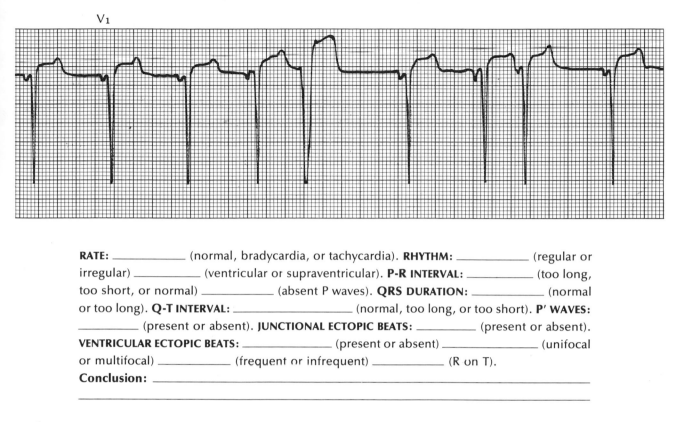

RATE: _____ (normal, bradycardia, or tachycardia). **RHYTHM:** _____ (regular or irregular) _____ (ventricular or supraventricular). **P-R INTERVAL:** _____ (too long, too short, or normal) _____ (absent P waves). **QRS DURATION:** _____ (normal or too long). **Q-T INTERVAL:** _____ (normal, too long, or too short). **P' WAVES:** _____ (present or absent). **JUNCTIONAL ECTOPIC BEATS:** _____ (present or absent).
VENTRICULAR ECTOPIC BEATS: _____ (present or absent) _____ (unifocal or multifocal) _____ (frequent or infrequent) _____ (R on T).
Conclusion: _____
_____

ANALYSIS

RATE: 80/min. (normal). **RHYTHM:** irregular and supraventricular. **P-R INTERVAL:** 0.09 sec. (too short). **QRS DURATION:** 0.06 sec. (normal). **Q-T INTERVAL:** 0.37 sec. (normal). **P' WAVES:** present. **JUNCTIONAL ECTOPIC BEATS:** absent. **VENTRICULAR ECTOPIC BEATS:** absent. **Conclusion:** Two PACs in this tracing are both followed by a reciprocating mechanism. The fourth P wave is premature and of a different morphology from the preceding P waves. It is followed by an atrial echo beat (in the T wave). The ventricular response (reciprocal beat) is conducted with LBBB aberration. The same sequence evolves with the next PAC (third P from the end). However, this time the reciprocal beat is conducted normally.

EXERCISE 8-4

I   II   III

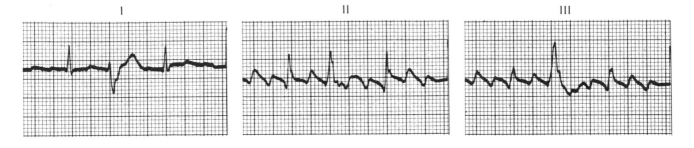

V₁

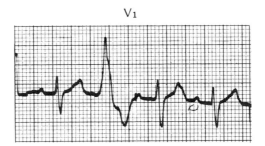

Simultaneous recordings.

RATE: _____ (normal, bradycardia, or tachycardia). **RHYTHM:** _____ (regular or irregular) _____ (ventricular or supraventricular). **P-R INTERVAL:** _____ (too long, too short, or normal) _____ (absent P waves). **QRS DURATION:** _____ (normal or too long). **Q-T INTERVAL:** _____ (normal, too long, or too short). **P′ WAVES:** _____ (present or absent). **JUNCTIONAL ECTOPIC BEATS:** _____ (present or absent).

VENTRICULAR ECTOPIC BEATS: _____ (present or absent) _____ (unifocal or multifocal) _____ (frequent or infrequent) _____ (R on T).

Conclusion: _____

_____

ANALYSIS

RATE: 100-110/min. (tachycardia). RHYTHM: irregular and supraventricular. P-R INTERVAL: absent P waves. QRS DURATION: 0.10 sec. (normal). Q-T INTERVAL: 0.32 sec. (normal). P′ WAVES: present. JUNCTIONAL ECTOPIC BEATS: absent. VENTRICULAR ECTOPIC BEATS: absent.

Conclusion: This is atrial flutter with 3:1 and 2:1 A-V conduction. In this case when conduction is 2:1, it is aberrant. The limb leads reflect LPH aberrancy, and lead V₁ reflects RBBB aberrancy. Therefore, when the conduction ratio is 2:1, the impulse is conducted only through the anterior fascicle of the left bundle. Note that the right axis deviation is picked up only in lead I. The atrial flutter waves are seen only in the inferior leads II and III. Lead I resembles atrial fibrillation, and lead V₁ looks like a sinus rhythm with first-degree heart block.

EXERCISE 8-5

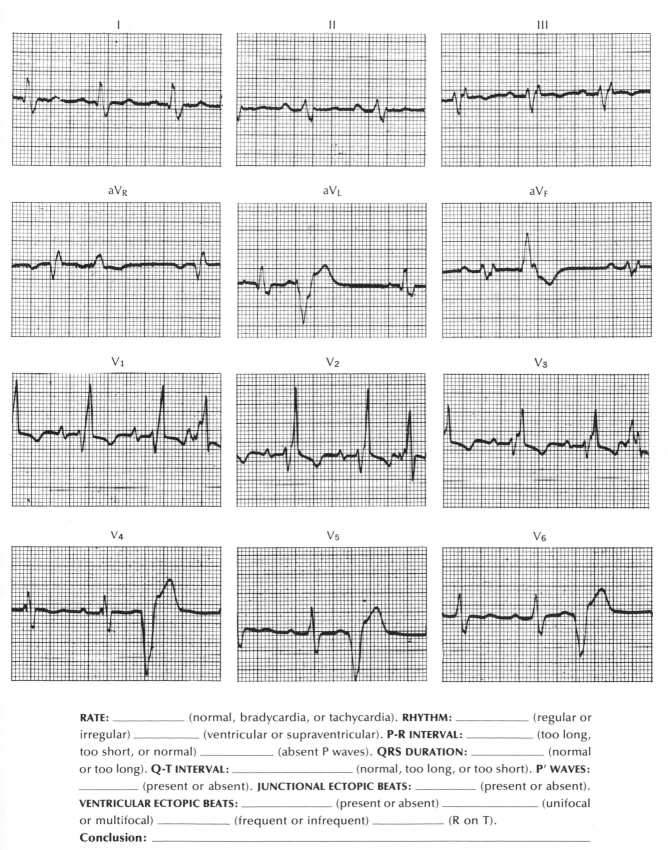

RATE: _____ (normal, bradycardia, or tachycardia). **RHYTHM:** _____ (regular or irregular) _____ (ventricular or supraventricular). **P-R INTERVAL:** _____ (too long, too short, or normal) _____ (absent P waves). **QRS DURATION:** _____ (normal or too long). **Q-T INTERVAL:** _____ (normal, too long, or too short). **P' WAVES:** _____ (present or absent). **JUNCTIONAL ECTOPIC BEATS:** _____ (present or absent). **VENTRICULAR ECTOPIC BEATS:** _____ (present or absent) _____ (unifocal or multifocal) _____ (frequent or infrequent) _____ (R on T).

Conclusion: _____

_____

ANALYSIS

RATE: 75/min. (normal). **RHYTHM:** irregular and supraventricular. **P-R INTERVAL:** 0.20 sec. (normal). **QRS DURATION:** 0.16 sec. (too long). **Q-T INTERVAL:** 0.42 sec. (too long). **P′ WAVES:** present. **JUNCTIONAL ECTOPIC BEATS:** absent. **VENTRICULAR ECTOPIC BEATS:** absent. **Conclusion:** The broad, premature beat seen in aV$_F$ is unquestionably the result of a PAC when seen in lead V$_1$. In this patient the P′ wave could only be seen in the right chest leads. It is important to search not only the limb leads but the precordial leads as well before you say that P waves or P′ waves are not present. Sometimes P waves are not seen in the conventional leads at all but are picked up in V$_3$R, an S$_5$, or a CR connection.

EXERCISE 8-6

V₁

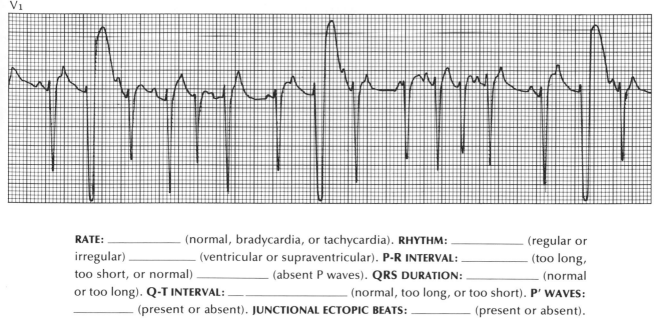

RATE: _____ (normal, bradycardia, or tachycardia). **RHYTHM:** _____ (regular or irregular) _____ (ventricular or supraventricular). **P-R INTERVAL:** _____ (too long, too short, or normal) _____ (absent P waves). **QRS DURATION:** _____ (normal or too long). **Q-T INTERVAL:** _____ (normal, too long, or too short). **P' WAVES:** _____ (present or absent). **JUNCTIONAL ECTOPIC BEATS:** _____ (present or absent). **VENTRICULAR ECTOPIC BEATS:** _____ (present or absent) _____ (unifocal or multifocal) _____ (frequent or infrequent) _____ (R on T).
Conclusion: _____

ANALYSIS

RATE: 150/min. (tachycardia). **RHYTHM:** irregular and supraventricular. **P-R INTERVAL:** difficult to determine P. **QRS DURATION:** 0.08 and 0.13 sec. (normal and too long). **Q-T INTERVAL:** varies. **P' WAVES:** present. **JUNCTIONAL ECTOPIC BEATS:** perhaps. **VENTRICULAR ECTOPIC BEATS:** absent.

Conclusion: The underlying arrhythmia in this tracing is chaotic atrial tachycardia (multifocal PACs). The broad complexes are supraventricular, conducted with LBBB aberration. Notice the r waves of the three complexes in question. They are narrow, reflecting initial activation of the anterior wall of the right ventricle as is sometimes seen in LBBB.

V₁

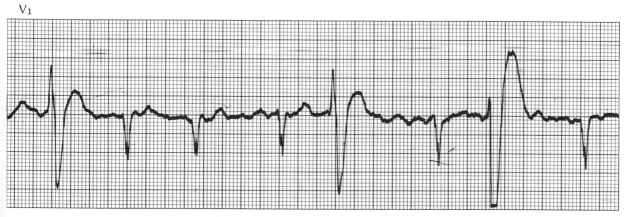

In the figure above, atrial fibrillation is the underlying arrhythmia. The three broad complexes resemble the ones at the top of the page. However, in this case the initial r waves are broad (beyond 0.03 sec.). The odds now are heavily in favor of right ventricular ectopy.

EXERCISE 8-7

II

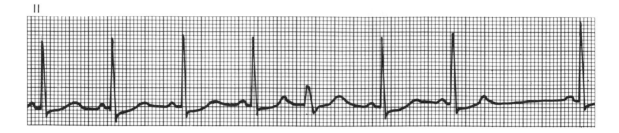

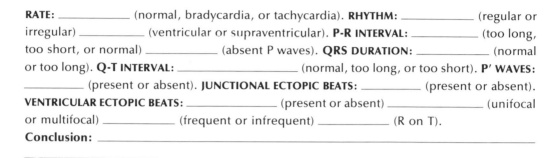

RATE: _____ (normal, bradycardia, or tachycardia). **RHYTHM:** _____ (regular or irregular) _____ (ventricular or supraventricular). **P-R INTERVAL:** _____ (too long, too short, or normal) _____ (absent P waves). **QRS DURATION:** _____ (normal or too long). **Q-T INTERVAL:** _____ (normal, too long, or too short). **P' WAVES:** _____ (present or absent). **JUNCTIONAL ECTOPIC BEATS:** _____ (present or absent). **VENTRICULAR ECTOPIC BEATS:** _____ (present or absent) _____ (unifocal or multifocal) _____ (frequent or infrequent) _____ (R on T). **Conclusion:** _____

ANALYSIS

RATE: 80/min. (normal). **RHYTHM:** irregular and supraventricular. **P-R INTERVAL:** 0.12 sec. (normal; constant). **QRS DURATION:** 0.08 sec. (normal). **Q-T INTERVAL:** 0.40 sec. (too long). **P' WAVES:** present. **JUNCTIONAL ECTOPIC BEATS:** absent. **VENTRICULAR ECTOPIC BEATS:** absent.

Conclusion: An abnormal complex and a pause are very apparent in this tracing. If you do not examine the tracing closely, you may decide that you have here a PVC and, later in the tracing, a sinus exit block. However, even to the casual observer it should be apparent that the broad ventricular complex is not followed by a full compensatory pause, indicating premature activation of the sinus node. A comparison of the T wave morphology reveals two P' waves in hiding. The T wave after the fourth complex is taller and more peaked than the dominant T waves. This is also seen in the T wave after the second-from-last complex. The first P' wave is followed by aberrant ventricular conduction; the last P' wave is not conducted at all, or perhaps it incompletely penetrates the A-V junction.

The change in cycle length due to the PAC is the cause of this ventricular aberration. As the coupling interval shortens, the impulse becomes more likely to meet with incompletely repolarized tissues during its spread through the His-Purkinje system.

EXERCISE 8-8

II

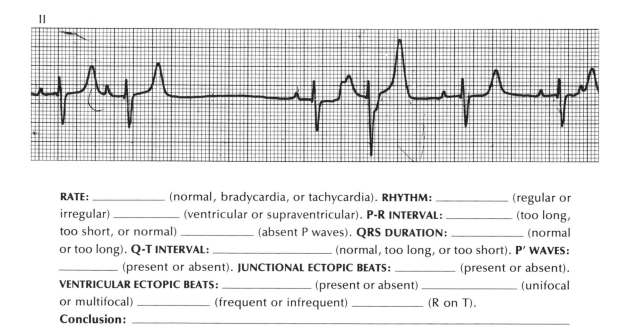

RATE: _____ (normal, bradycardia, or tachycardia). **RHYTHM:** _____ (regular or irregular) _____ (ventricular or supraventricular). **P-R INTERVAL:** _____ (too long, too short, or normal) _____ (absent P waves). **QRS DURATION:** _____ (normal or too long). **Q-T INTERVAL:** _____ (normal, too long, or too short). **P' WAVES:** _____ (present or absent). **JUNCTIONAL ECTOPIC BEATS:** _____ (present or absent). **VENTRICULAR ECTOPIC BEATS:** _____ (present or absent) _____ (unifocal or multifocal) _____ (frequent or infrequent) _____ (R on T).
Conclusion: _____

ANALYSIS

RATE: 60/min. (normal). **RHYTHM:** irregular and supraventricular. **P-R INTERVAL:** 0.22 sec. (too long; constant). **QRS DURATION:** 0.10 sec. (normal). **Q-T INTERVAL:** 0.46 sec. (too long). **P' WAVES:** present. **JUNCTIONAL ECTOPIC BEATS:** absent. **VENTRICULAR ECTOPIC BEATS:** absent.

Conclusion: The second P wave in this tracing is premature and of a different morphology from the first. A nonconducted P' wave is present in the T wave preceding the pause. The next PAC (deforming the T wave of the third complex) is followed by aberrant ventricular conduction (LBBB). Two factors are causing this aberrant beat: a short coupling interval and the duration of the preceding cycle. A long preceding cycle causes a broader action potential, which would increase the chances of a premature supraventricular impulse's meeting with tissues that are still repolarizing.

The third P' wave in this tracing is so premature that it is not conducted at all (not shown). This PAC occurs just before the last T wave.

EXERCISE 8-9

II

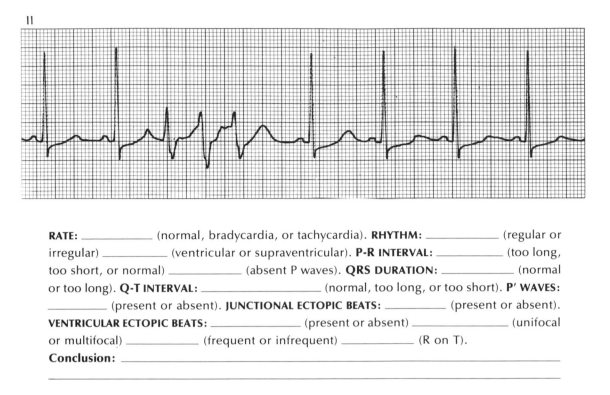

RATE: _____ (normal, bradycardia, or tachycardia). **RHYTHM:** _____ (regular or irregular) _____ (ventricular or supraventricular). **P-R INTERVAL:** _____ (too long, too short, or normal) _____ (absent P waves). **QRS DURATION:** _____ (normal or too long). **Q-T INTERVAL:** _____ (normal, too long, or too short). **P' WAVES:** _____ (present or absent). **JUNCTIONAL ECTOPIC BEATS:** _____ (present or absent).
VENTRICULAR ECTOPIC BEATS: _____ (present or absent) _____ (unifocal or multifocal) _____ (frequent or infrequent) _____ (R on T).
Conclusion: _____
_____

ANALYSIS

RATE: 78/min. (normal). **RHYTHM:** irregular and supraventricular. **P-R INTERVAL:** 0.15 sec. (normal; constant). **QRS DURATION:** 0.08 sec. (normal). **Q-T INTERVAL:** 0.52 sec. (too long). **P' WAVES:** present. **JUNCTIONAL ECTOPIC BEATS:** absent. **VENTRICULAR ECTOPIC BEATS:** absent.

Conclusion: The peaked T wave in front of the burst of tachycardia is a telltale sign of a hidden P' wave. This P' is followed by three aberrantly conducted beats, probably an A-V nodal reciprocating mechanism.

EXERCISE 8-10

V₁

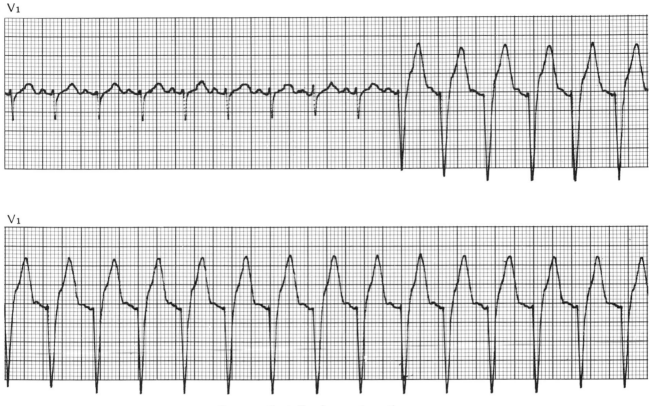

Same patient. Tracings not continuous.

RATE: _____ (normal, bradycardia, or tachycardia). **RHYTHM:** _____ (regular or irregular) _____ (ventricular or supraventricular). **P-R INTERVAL:** _____ (too long, too short, or normal) _____ (absent P waves). **QRS DURATION:** _____ (normal or too long). **Q-T INTERVAL:** _____ (normal, too long, or too short). **P′ WAVES:** _____ (present or absent). **JUNCTIONAL ECTOPIC BEATS:** _____ (present or absent). **VENTRICULAR ECTOPIC BEATS:** _____ (present or absent) _____ (unifocal or multifocal) _____ (frequent or infrequent) _____ (R on T).
Conclusion: _____
_____

ANALYSIS

RATE: 130/min. (tachycardia). **RHYTHM:** regular and supraventricular. **P-R INTERVAL:** 0.12 sec. (normal). **QRS DURATION:** 0.07 and 0.12 sec. (normal and too long). **Q-T INTERVAL:** 0.28 sec. (normal). **P′ WAVES:** questionable. **JUNCTIONAL ECTOPIC BEATS:** absent. **VENTRICULAR ECTOPIC BEATS:** absent.

Conclusion: In this tracing we see the onset of LBBB. The bottom tracing could easily be mistaken for ventricular tachycardia. However, with the onset in view, there is no question that this is a supraventricular tachycardia.

Whenever the sinus rate is 130-170/min. you should always suspect a hidden P wave and therefore an atrial ectopic rate of twice as much. If you take the midpoint between two apparent P waves, you will find that if there were a hidden P′ wave, it would coincide with the T wave. When a P′ wave occurs in every T wave, it will distort differently each time, since it is not really part of the mechanism of ventricular repolarization. Such is the case here. The T waves are all different, perhaps distorted by a hidden P′, in which case this would be atrial flutter or tachycardia with 2:1 A-V conduction. Carotid sinus pressure may confirm the diagnosis.

Clinically, this ventricular rate cannot long be tolerated by an already ischemic heart and should be converted to a normal sinus rhythm.

EXERCISE 8-11

MCL₁

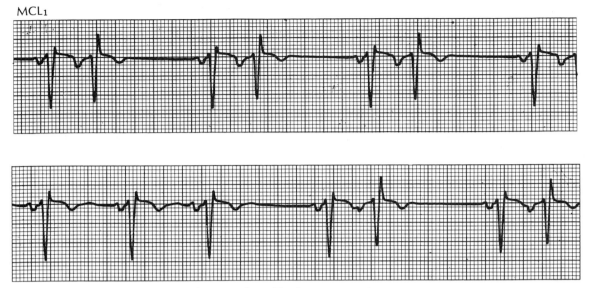

Same patient. Tracings not continuous.

RATE: _____ (normal, bradycardia, or tachycardia). **RHYTHM:** _____ (regular or irregular) _____ (ventricular or supraventricular). **P-R INTERVAL:** _____ (too long, too short, or normal) _____ (absent P waves). **QRS DURATION:** _____ (normal or too long). **Q-T INTERVAL:** _____ (normal, too long, or too short). **P′ WAVES:** _____ (present or absent). **JUNCTIONAL ECTOPIC BEATS:** _____ (present or absent). **VENTRICULAR ECTOPIC BEATS:** _____ (present or absent) _____ (unifocal or multifocal) _____ (frequent or infrequent) _____ (R on T). **Conclusion:** _____

ANALYSIS

RATE: 70/min. (normal). **RHYTHM:** irregular and supraventricular. **P-R INTERVAL:** 0.13 sec. (normal; constant). **QRS DURATION:** 0.12 sec. (too long). **Q-T INTERVAL:** 0.42 sec. (too long). **P′ WAVES:** present. **JUNCTIONAL ECTOPIC BEATS:** absent. **VENTRICULAR ECTOPIC BEATS:** absent.

Conclusion: The genesis of the bigeminal rhythm in the first tracing becomes more readily apparent when you look at the second tracing from the same patient, in which the first two complexes are normal sinus in origin. These are followed by a PAC that appears to initiate bigeminal PACs, all of which are conducted with more RBBB than is already present in the dominant rhythm.

EXERCISE 8-12

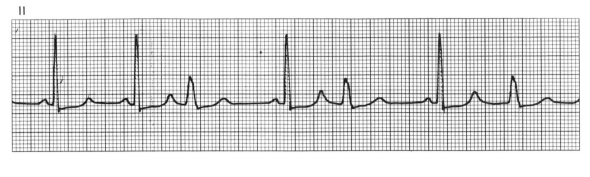

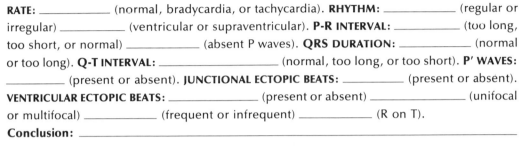

RATE: _____ (normal, bradycardia, or tachycardia). **RHYTHM:** _____ (regular or irregular) _____ (ventricular or supraventricular). **P-R INTERVAL:** _____ (too long, too short, or normal) _____ (absent P waves). **QRS DURATION:** _____ (normal or too long). **Q-T INTERVAL:** _____ (normal, too long, or too short). **P' WAVES:** _____ (present or absent). **JUNCTIONAL ECTOPIC BEATS:** _____ (present or absent). **VENTRICULAR ECTOPIC BEATS:** _____ (present or absent) _____ (unifocal or multifocal) _____ (frequent or infrequent) _____ (R on T). **Conclusion:** _____

_____

ANALYSIS

RATE: 68/min. (normal). **RHYTHM:** irregular and supraventricular. **P-R INTERVAL:** 0.16 sec. (normal; constant). **QRS DURATION:** 0.07 sec. (normal). **Q-T INTERVAL:** 0.42 sec. (too long). **P' WAVES:** present. **JUNCTIONAL ECTOPIC BEATS:** absent. **VENTRICULAR ECTOPIC BEATS:** absent.

Conclusion: Here again, as in the preceding exercise, the bigeminal rhythm is due to PACs conducted aberrantly through the ventricles. The first two complexes are normally conducted sinus beats; afterward a change in the shape of the T wave is noted, indicative of a hidden P' wave. The impulse is conducted aberrantly because of the short coupling interval along with the abrupt change in cycle length.

EXERCISE 8-13

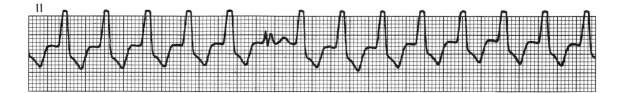

RATE: _____ (normal, bradycardia, or tachycardia). **RHYTHM:** _____ (regular or irregular) _____ (ventricular or supraventricular). **P-R INTERVAL:** _____ (too long, too short, or normal) _____ (absent P waves). **QRS DURATION:** _____ (normal or too long). **Q-T INTERVAL:** _____ (normal, too long, or too short). **P′ WAVES:** _____ (present or absent). **JUNCTIONAL ECTOPIC BEATS:** _____ (present or absent).

VENTRICULAR ECTOPIC BEATS: _____ (present or absent) _____ (unifocal or multifocal) _____ (frequent or infrequent) _____ (R on T).

Conclusion: _____

_____

ANALYSIS

RATE: 135/min. in both tracings (tachycardia). RHYTHM: regular and probably ventricular. **P-R INTERVAL:** not applicable. **QRS DURATION:** 0.12 sec. (too long). **Q-T INTERVAL:** 0.36 and 0.32 sec. (too long). **P′ WAVES:** absent. **JUNCTIONAL ECTOPIC BEATS:** absent. **VENTRICULAR ECTOPIC BEATS:** present, premature, frequent, and unifocal.

Conclusion: There is a Dressler beat (ventricular fusion beat) present in this tracing, as reflected in the narrower complex of lesser amplitude. This could indicate one of two possibilities. The first is that during ventricular tachycardia, a sinus impulse partially captured the ventricles; that is, a sinus impulse has found the A-V junction nonrefractory and has descended and fused with the ectopic activity. The second possibility is that a supraventricular tachycardia is in effect and a ventricular ectopic beat has discharged at the same time, causing a fusion of the supraventricular pacemaker vector and the ventricular ectopic vector. Thus the arrhythmia may be either ventricular or supraventricular with aberration. Unless there are morphological clues in lead V_1 or V_6 strongly favoring aberration, this arrhythmia should be treated aggressively as a ventricular tachycardia. Aberrancy should never be postulated without proof.

EXERCISE 8-14

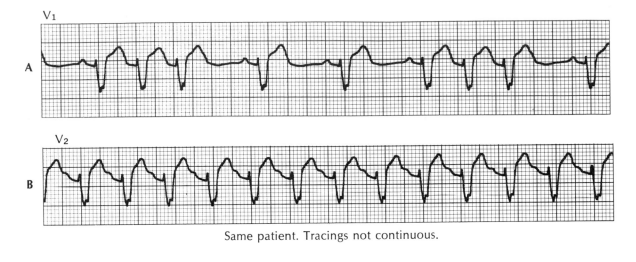

V₁

A

V₂

B

Same patient. Tracings not continuous.

RATE: _____ (normal, bradycardia, or tachycardia). **RHYTHM:** _____ (regular or irregular) _____ (ventricular or supraventricular). **P-R INTERVAL:** _____ (too long, too short, or normal) _____ (absent P waves). **QRS DURATION:** _____ (normal or too long). **Q-T INTERVAL:** _____ (normal, too long, or too short). **P' WAVES:** _____ (present or absent). **JUNCTIONAL ECTOPIC BEATS:** _____ (present or absent).

VENTRICULAR ECTOPIC BEATS: _____ (present or absent) _____ (unifocal or multifocal) _____ (frequent or infrequent) _____ (R on T).

Conclusion: _____

_____

ANALYSIS

RATE: *A*, 90/ min. (normal); *B*, 130/min. (tachycardia). RHYTHM: *A*, irregular; *B*, regular; supraventricular in both. P-R INTERVAL: 0.16 sec. (normal; constant). QRS DURATION: 0.12 sec. (too long). Q-T INTERVAL: 0.32 sec. (normal). P' WAVES: absent. JUNCTIONAL ECTOPIC BEATS: present and premature. VENTRICULAR ECTOPIC BEATS: absent.

Conclusion: A look at the isolated extrasystoles leaves no doubt as to the origin of this tachycardia. The dominant rhythm in the first tracing is a sinus rhythm with LBBB. Premature junctional beats are present, which are paired and conducted with the same BBB pattern as the sinus-conducted beats. Identical complexes are seen in the tachycardia, which resemble those of ventricular tachycardia because of their broad morphology but which are those of sinus tachycardia with LBBB.

EXERCISE 8-15

II

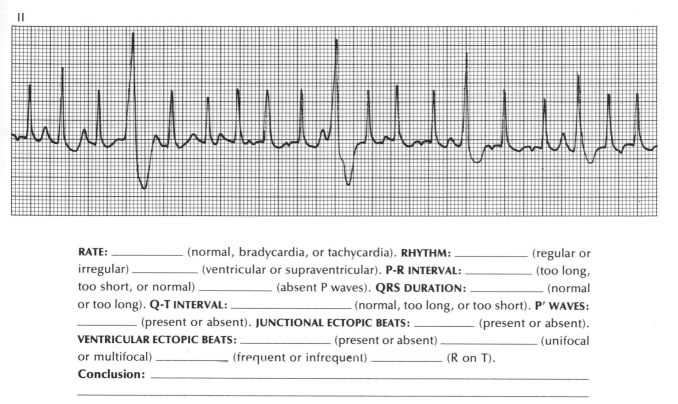

RATE: _____ (normal, bradycardia, or tachycardia). **RHYTHM:** _____ (regular or irregular) _____ (ventricular or supraventricular). **P-R INTERVAL:** _____ (too long, too short, or normal) _____ (absent P waves). **QRS DURATION:** _____ (normal or too long). **Q-T INTERVAL:** _____ (normal, too long, or too short). **P' WAVES:** _____ (present or absent). **JUNCTIONAL ECTOPIC BEATS:** _____ (present or absent). **VENTRICULAR ECTOPIC BEATS:** _____ (present or absent) _____ (unifocal or multifocal) _____ (frequent or infrequent) _____ (R on T).
Conclusion: _____
_____

ANALYSIS

RATE: 170/min. (tachycardia). **RHYTHM:** irregular and supraventricular with ventricular. **P-R INTERVAL:** absent P waves. **QRS DURATION:** 0.08 sec. (normal). **Q-T INTERVAL:** varies. **P' WAVES:** present. **JUNCTIONAL ECTOPIC BEATS:** present. **VENTRICULAR ECTOPIC BEATS:** present, frequent, and unifocal.

Conclusion: There is chaotic atrial activity with junctional and atrial ectopics at a very rapid rate in this tracing. This rapid ventricular rate is, of course, the main concern. The tall, broad complexes are ventricular ectopics. We know this because some of them are fusion beats (second complex from the beginning and the third and sixth from the end). When the underlying arrhythmia is decidedly supraventricular in origin, the only possible way a fusion beat could occur is with the help of a ventricular ectopic mechanism. The question of aberrancy is also negated because other complexes with shorter coupling intervals and preceding longer cycles are conducted normally (for example, the seventh complex).

To review, we know that there are PVCs in this tracing because of fusion beats and normal conduction with shorter cycles.

EXERCISE 8-16

V₁

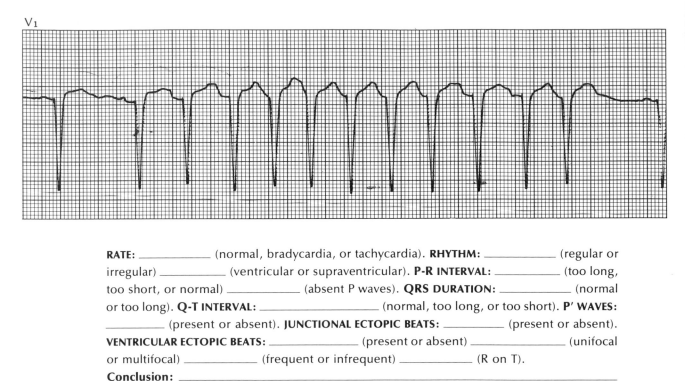

RATE: _____ (normal, bradycardia, or tachycardia). **RHYTHM:** _____ (regular or irregular) _____ (ventricular or supraventricular). **P-R INTERVAL:** _____ (too long, too short, or normal) _____ (absent P waves). **QRS DURATION:** _____ (normal or too long). **Q-T INTERVAL:** _____ (normal, too long, or too short). **P′ WAVES:** _____ (present or absent). **JUNCTIONAL ECTOPIC BEATS:** _____ (present or absent). **VENTRICULAR ECTOPIC BEATS:** _____ (present or absent) _____ (unifocal or multifocal) _____ (frequent or infrequent) _____ (R on T). **Conclusion:** _____
_____

ANALYSIS

RATE: 130/min. (tachycardia). **RHYTHM:** irregular and supraventricular. **P-R INTERVAL:** 0.13 sec. (normal). **QRS DURATION:** 0.12 sec. (too long). **Q-T INTERVAL:** varies. **P′ WAVES:** present. **JUNCTIONAL ECTOPIC BEATS:** present. **VENTRICULAR ECTOPIC BEATS:** absent.

Conclusion: This is a paroxysmal supraventricular tachycardia initiated by a PAC (second P wave). There is an underlying BBB, which might cause diagnostic problems if the onset of the tachycardia is not seen or if the observer does not know that the patient had BBB.

EXERCISE 8-17

V₁

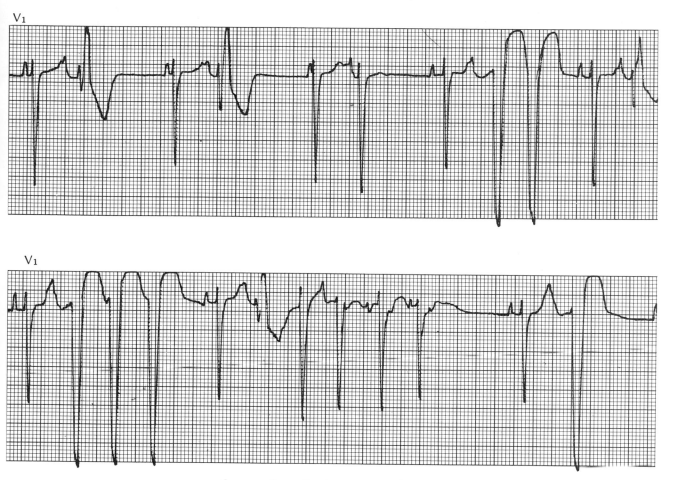

V₁

Same patient. Tracings not continuous.

RATE: _____ (normal, bradycardia, or tachycardia). **RHYTHM:** _____ (regular or irregular) _____ (ventricular or supraventricular). **P-R INTERVAL:** _____ (too long, too short, or normal) _____ (absent P waves). **QRS DURATION:** _____ (normal or too long). **Q-T INTERVAL:** _____ (normal, too long, or too short). **P′ WAVES:** _____ (present or absent). **JUNCTIONAL ECTOPIC BEATS:** _____ (present or absent).
VENTRICULAR ECTOPIC BEATS: _____ (present or absent) _____ (unifocal or multifocal) _____ (frequent or infrequent) _____ (R on T).
Conclusion: _____ _____

ANALYSIS

RATE: 90-150/min. (tachycardia). RHYTHM: irregular and supraventricular. P-R INTERVAL: 0.12 sec. (normal). QRS DURATION: 0.10 sec. (normal). Q-T INTERVAL: varies. P′ WAVES: present. JUNCTIONAL ECTOPIC BEATS: absent. VENTRICULAR ECTOPIC BEATS: absent.
Conclusion: The PACs are very evident in this tracing, distorting the T waves. They are conducted with both RBBB and LBBB aberration.

In the bottom tracing the first beat is sinus conducted. There is a P′ wave in the T wave, which initiates a burst of supraventricular tachycardia. The first three complexes of the tachycardia are conducted with LBBB aberration. The fourth beat is conducted normally and then with RBBB aberration. The remainder of the tachycardia is conducted normally and with incomplete LBBB aberration.

213

EXERCISE 8-18

V₁

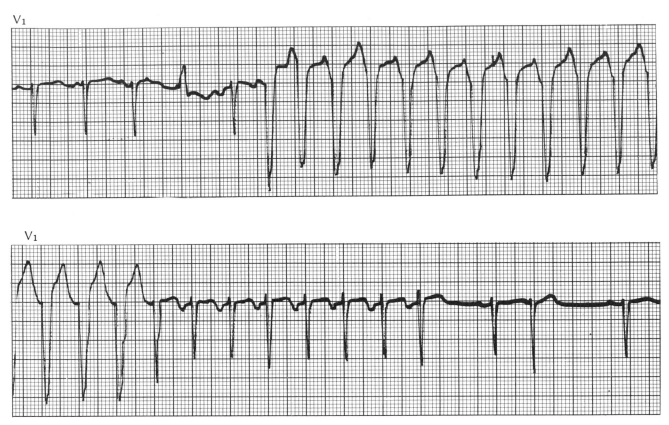

V₁

Same patient. Tracings not continuous.

RATE: _____ (normal, bradycardia, or tachycardia). **RHYTHM:** _____ (regular or irregular) _____ (ventricular or supraventricular). **P-R INTERVAL:** _____ (too long, too short, or normal) _____ (absent P waves). **QRS DURATION:** _____ (normal or too long). **Q-T INTERVAL:** _____ (normal, too long, or too short). **P' WAVES:** _____ (present or absent). **JUNCTIONAL ECTOPIC BEATS:** _____ (present or absent). **VENTRICULAR ECTOPIC BEATS:** _____ (present or absent) _____ (unifocal or multifocal) _____ (frequent or infrequent) _____ (R on T). **Conclusion:** _____

_____

ANALYSIS

RATE: 100-150/min. (tachycardia). RHYTHM: irregular and supraventricular. P-R INTERVAL: 0.14 sec. (normal). QRS DURATION: 0.08 and 0.12 sec. (normal and too long). Q-T INTERVAL: varies. P' WAVES: present. JUNCTIONAL ECTOPIC BEATS: present. VENTRICULAR ECTOPIC BEATS: absent.

Conclusion: This is a paroxysmal supraventricular tachycardia with LBBB aberration. The first beat is sinus, followed by two premature junctional ectopics (note the short P'-R interval). The P' wave in the third T is probably an atrial echo beat. It is followed by a reciprocal beat of RBBB configuration. This begins a rapid A-V nodal reentry mechanism, which is clearly seen as it ends in normal conduction in the second tracing.

EXERCISE 8-19

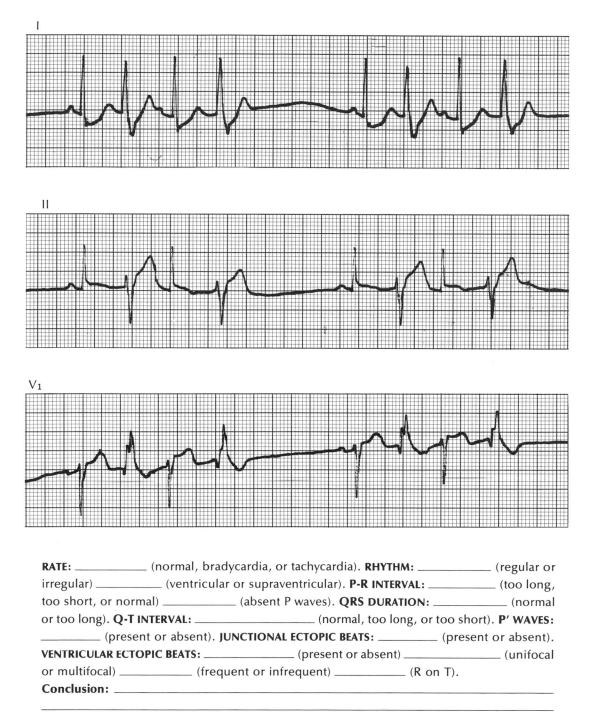

I

II

V₁

RATE: _____ (normal, bradycardia, or tachycardia). **RHYTHM:** _____ (regular or irregular) _____ (ventricular or supraventricular). **P-R INTERVAL:** _____ (too long, too short, or normal) _____ (absent P waves). **QRS DURATION:** _____ (normal or too long). **Q-T INTERVAL:** _____ (normal, too long, or too short). **P' WAVES:** _____ (present or absent). **JUNCTIONAL ECTOPIC BEATS:** _____ (present or absent). **VENTRICULAR ECTOPIC BEATS:** _____ (present or absent) _____ (unifocal or multifocal) _____ (frequent or infrequent) _____ (R on T).
Conclusion: _____
_____

ANALYSIS

RATE: approximately 80/min. (normal). RHYTHM: irregular and supraventricular. P-R INTERVAL: 0.14 sec. (normal). QRS DURATION: 0.08 and 0.14 sec. (normal and too long). Q-T INTERVAL: varies. P' WAVES: present. JUNCTIONAL ECTOPIC BEATS: present. VENTRICULAR ECTOPIC BEATS: absent.

Conclusion: This patient had bursts of supraventricular tachycardia, which always terminated after 3 beats. In lead I every other beat is broadened by an s wave. This is the typical morphology of RBBB in leads I and V_6. Lead II indicates that the broad beats have LAD, reflective of LAH. In lead V_1 the broad beats in question are primarily positive. P' waves can be seen in all three leads. They are conducted with bifascicular block (LAH and RBBB aberration).

EXERCISE 8-20

V₁

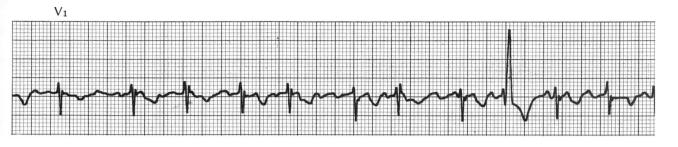

RATE: _____ (normal, bradycardia, or tachycardia). **RHYTHM:** _____ (regular or irregular) _____ (ventricular or supraventricular). **P-R INTERVAL:** _____ (too long, too short, or normal) _____ (absent P waves). **QRS DURATION:** _____ (normal or too long). **Q-T INTERVAL:** _____ (normal, too long, or too short). **P' WAVES:** _____ (present or absent). **JUNCTIONAL ECTOPIC BEATS:** _____ (present or absent). **VENTRICULAR ECTOPIC BEATS:** _____ (present or absent) _____ (unifocal or multifocal) _____ (frequent or infrequent) _____ (R on T).

Conclusion: _____

_____

ANALYSIS

RATE: approximately 110/min. (tachycardia). RHYTHM: irregular and supraventricular.
P-R INTERVAL: absent P waves. QRS DURATION: 0.08 sec. (normal). Q-T INTERVAL: difficult
to determine. P' WAVES: absent. JUNCTIONAL ECTOPIC BEATS: absent. VENTRICULAR ECTOPIC
BEATS: absent.

Conclusion: This is atrial fibrillation with one aberrantly conducted beat (RBBB). The broad complex toward the end of the tracing has the classical RBBB pattern, as seen in lead V₁. That is, initial forces are normal, and terminal forces are late and to the right.

CHAPTER 9

PATTERNS IN MYOCARDIAL INFARCTION

The exercises in this chapter are designed to give you experience in determining the presence and location of a myocardial infarction (MI) from the twelve-lead ECG. A full explanation of patho- and electrophysiology can be found in the textbooks listed in the general section of the references. The following is a brief review.

When a coronary artery is completely occluded, the muscle supplied by that vessel will become ischemic. Within minutes the fibers in the center will become nonfunctional and then necrotic. Thus, from the center of the infarcted area outward there will be necrosis, nonfunctional tissue, and then ischemic tissue. In the evolving myocardial infarction, the area of dead fibers enlarges because the marginal fibers succumb from the prolonged ischemia. At the same time the collateral circulation improves, and the outer rim of nonfunctional tissue becomes smaller and smaller. When the initial area of infarction is large, it may take 2 or 3 weeks for all of the nonfunctional area to become functional again or to become necrotic.

These progressive changes are reflected from day to day in the ECG as follows. The acute stage, where nonfunctional tissue is present, will produce a current of injury and S-T segment elevation, which is typically coved upward. The irreversible structural changes resulting from tissue death are reflected by abnormal Q waves, which will persist after the S-T and T changes have resolved. The S-T segment will gradually lower to T wave inversion (ischemia), which is typically symmetrical and arrow shaped. The abnormal Q wave is diagnostic, while S-T and T changes are supportive. These are termed "indicative changes," and all three may be present at the same time in any one lead.

Reciprocal changes will be seen in leads reflecting the surface on the side of the heart opposite to the infarct. For example, when there is S-T elevation in the inferior leads (II, III, and aV_F), there may be S-T depression in leads V_1 to V_3, I, and aV_L, T wave inversion may have reciprocal heightening of the T wave in opposite leads, and abnormal Q waves will have reciprocal heightening of the R waves. Sometimes reciprocal changes are seen even before indicative ones.

The ECG signs of myocardial infarction confirm and support the clinical impression. One never proceeds on the ECG alone, nor does one make a diagnosis from a single tracing. There are other conditions that mimic the ECG of infarction but that do not evolve as does the myocardial infarction and that do not manifest clinically as does the myocardial infarction. Ventricular hypertrophy, Wolff-Parkinson-White syndrome, and diffuse myocardial disease are a few of the mimics. Then, too, a clinically certain myocardial infarction may demonstrate ECG signs of infarction only late or, rarely, not at all.

For the nurse in the critical care unit, knowing how to recognize the ECG signs of a fresh infarction is far more important than being able to determine the location. However, the latter is simply a matter of knowing which leads reflect which cardiac surfaces. Think of the heart as having inferior, lateral, and anterior surfaces (true posterior will be discussed separately under that exercise). The lateral and anterior surfaces are really superior. The leads are divided, for our purposes now, into inferior (II, III, and aV$_F$), and superior (V$_1$ to V$_6$, I, and aV$_L$). The leads whose positive electrode are at the left shoulder and left axillary region "look down" on the lateral wall (I, aV$_L$, V$_5$, and V$_6$). The anterior wall is just under leads V$_1$ to V$_4$. The inferior leads, of course, reflect the inferior, or diaphragmatic, surface.

As you proceed with the following exercises, keep reviewing the above information. Remember that you will be looking for S-T elevation, T wave inversion, and abnormal Q waves. A few of the mimics are included so that you can appreciate the differential diagnosis.

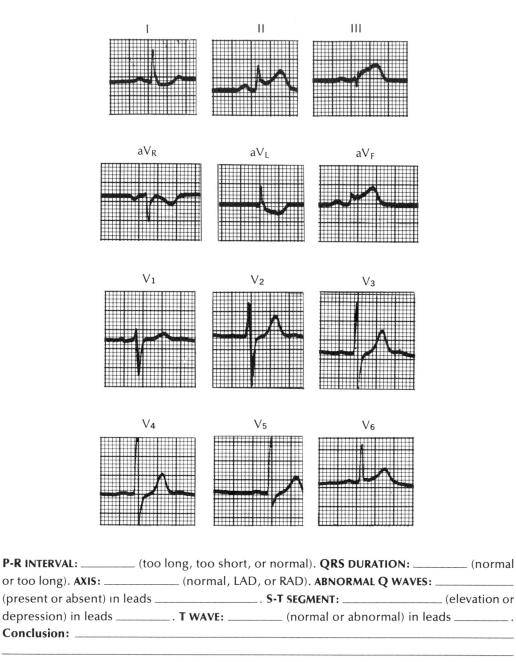

P-R INTERVAL: _____ (too long, too short, or normal). **QRS DURATION:** _____ (normal or too long). **AXIS:** _____ (normal, LAD, or RAD). **ABNORMAL Q WAVES:** _____ (present or absent) in leads _____ . **S-T SEGMENT:** _____ (elevation or depression) in leads _____ . **T WAVE:** _____ (normal or abnormal) in leads _____ .
Conclusion: _____

ANALYSIS

P-R INTERVAL: 0.16 sec. (normal). **QRS DURATION:** 0.08 sec. (normal). **AXIS:** normal. **S-T SEGMENT:** ↑ II, III, aV_F, and V_6; ↓ I. **T WAVE INVERSION:** aV_L. **ABNORMAL Q WAVES:** none.
Conclusion: This is an acute, inferior wall myocardial infarction with extension to the apex, and lateral wall ischemia. S-T elevation, indicating the acute phase of myocardial infarction, is seen in the leads that reflect the inferior wall of the heart (II, III, and aV_F). The S-T elevation in lead V_6 reflects involvement of the apex. The positive electrode of aV_L looks down on the lateral wall of the heart. The T wave in this tracing is inverted in that lead, indicating that the ischemic edge of the infarcted area extends to the lateral wall.

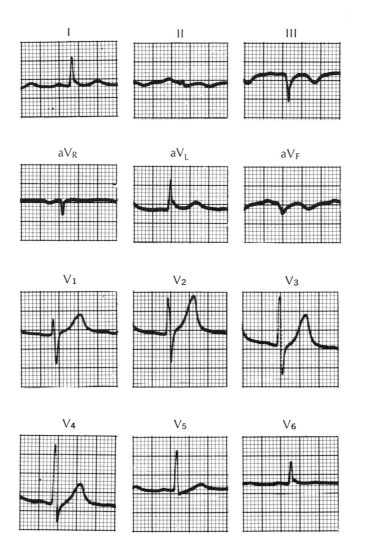

Eighteen days later (see figure above) you can see the evolving pattern of an inferior infarction. In the inferior leads where S-T elevation was previously present, the S-T segment has coved typically, and the T waves have inverted. There are now QS waves in leads II and aV_F. At this stage in the evolution of the infarction, the nonfunctional tissue, reflected by the previous S-T elevation, has either become necrotic (Q waves) or ischemic (T wave inversion).

EXERCISE 9-2

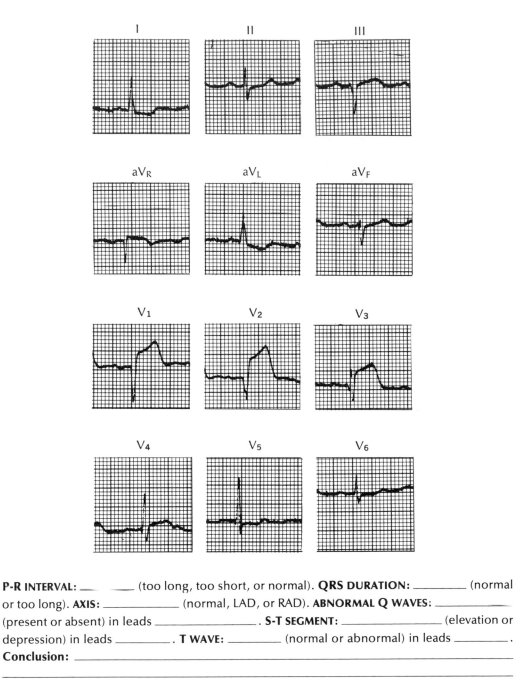

P-R INTERVAL: ___ ___ (too long, too short, or normal). **QRS DURATION:** _____ (normal or too long). **AXIS:** _____ (normal, LAD, or RAD). **ABNORMAL Q WAVES:** _____ (present or absent) in leads _____ . **S-T SEGMENT:** _____ (elevation or depression) in leads _____ . **T WAVE:** _____ (normal or abnormal) in leads _____ .
Conclusion: _____

ANALYSIS

P-R INTERVAL: 0.18 sec. (normal). **QRS DURATION:** 0.08 sec. (normal). **AXIS:** normal. **S-T SEGMENT:** ↑ V₁ to V₄; ↓ II. **T WAVE INVERSION:** I and aV_L. **ABNORMAL Q WAVES:** V₁ to V₃. **Conclusion:** This is an acute, anteroseptal myocardial infarction. A current of injury is seen in the leads over the septum (V₁ to V₃). Subtle signs of ischemia are present in leads that reflect the lateral wall (I, aV_L, V₅, and V₆). That is, there is lowering of the S-T segment and T waves in leads I, aV_L, V₅, and V₆.

EXERCISE 9-3

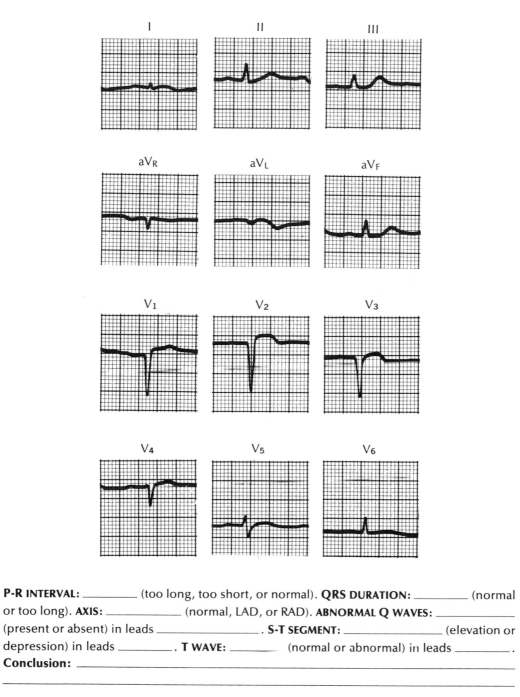

P-R INTERVAL: _____ (too long, too short, or normal). **QRS DURATION:** _____ (normal or too long). **AXIS:** _____ (normal, LAD, or RAD). **ABNORMAL Q WAVES:** _____ (present or absent) in leads _____ . **S-T SEGMENT:** _____ (elevation or depression) in leads _____ . **T WAVE:** _____ (normal or abnormal) in leads _____ .
Conclusion: _____

_____

ANALYSIS

P-R INTERVAL: 0.20 sec. (normal). **QRS DURATION:** 0.08 sec. (normal). **AXIS:** normal. **S-T SEGMENT:** ↑ V_1 to V_4. **T WAVE INVERSION:** I and aV_L. **ABNORMAL Q WAVES:** V_1 to V_4 and aV_L. **Conclusion:** This is an evolving, anteroseptal myocardial infarction with extension to the lateral wall. The S-T segments are still slightly elevated in the anterior chest leads (reflecting the anteroseptal area). There is evidence of extension to the lateral wall in the leads reflecting that surface. That is, there is coving of the S-T segment in leads V_5, V_6, I, and aV_L, with T wave inversion in leads I and aV_L. Note that the loss of normal septal forces is not only reflected by the absence of r waves from leads V_1 to V_4 but also in the absence of normal little q waves in leads I and V_6.

As the healing process continues, the T waves in the anterior precordial leads will invert and become symmetrical and arrow shaped. This may also be the case in the leads reflecting the lateral wall.

EXERCISE 9-4

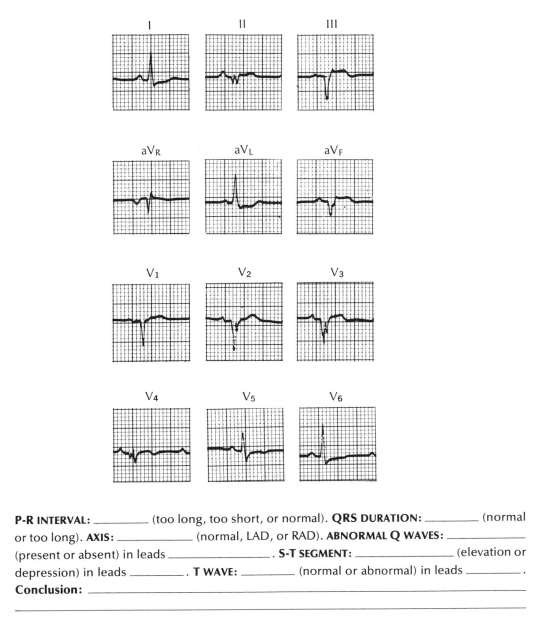

P-R INTERVAL: _____ (too long, too short, or normal). **QRS DURATION:** _____ (normal or too long). **AXIS:** _____ (normal, LAD, or RAD). **ABNORMAL Q WAVES:** _____ (present or absent) in leads _____ . **S-T SEGMENT:** _____ (elevation or depression) in leads _____ . **T WAVE:** _____ (normal or abnormal) in leads _____ .
Conclusion: _____

ANALYSIS

P-R INTERVAL: 0.12 sec. (normal). **QRS DURATION:** 0.09 sec. (normal). **AXIS:** LAD. **S-T SEGMENT:** ↑ II, III, aV$_F$, and V$_1$ to V$_3$. ↓ I and aV$_L$. **T WAVE INVERSION:** V$_4$ and V$_5$. **ABNORMAL Q WAVES:** II, III, aV$_F$, and V$_1$ to V$_4$.

Conclusion: In this ECG there is evidence for anteroseptal infarction of undetermined age. It could be recent or quite old, but it is not acute. The S-T elevation in the inferior leads, if it can be shown to be an evolving pattern in serial ECGs, is reflective of acute, inferior wall myocardial infarction. However, it should be mentioned that S-T elevation can persist for months and years in the presence of a ventricular aneurysm. Hence, you can see the importance of noting the evolving pattern before making the diagnosis of acute myocardial infarction.

EXERCISE 9-5

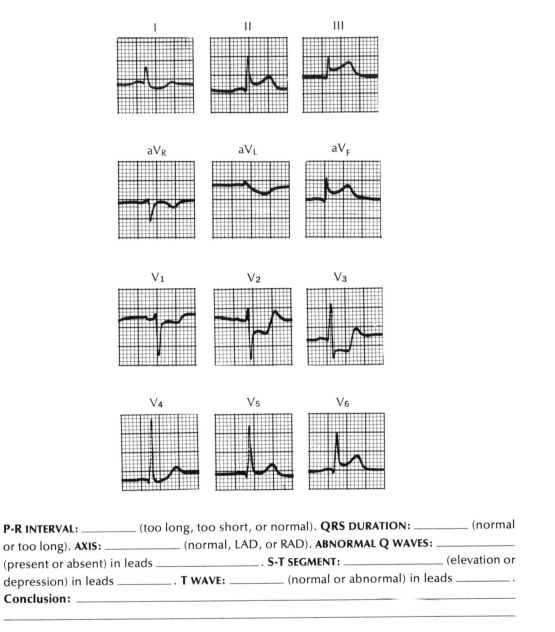

P-R INTERVAL: _____ (too long, too short, or normal). **QRS DURATION:** _____ (normal or too long). **AXIS:** _____ (normal, LAD, or RAD). **ABNORMAL Q WAVES:** _____ (present or absent) in leads _____ . **S-T SEGMENT:** _____ (elevation or depression) in leads _____ . **T WAVE:** _____ (normal or abnormal) in leads _____ .
Conclusion: _____

ANALYSIS

P-R INTERVAL: 0.12 sec. (normal). **QRS DURATION:** 0.08 sec. (normal). **AXIS:** normal. **S-T SEGMENT:** ↑ II, III, and aV_F; ↓ V_1 to V_3. **T WAVE INVERSION:** I and aV_L. **ABNORMAL Q WAVES:** absent.

Conclusion: This is an acute, inferior wall myocardial infarction. There is S-T segment elevation in the leads reflecting that wall of the heart. Reciprocal changes can be seen in leads V_1 to V_3. This myocardial infarction is probably in the hyperacute phase in that Q waves have not yet developed in the inferior leads.

EXERCISE 9-6

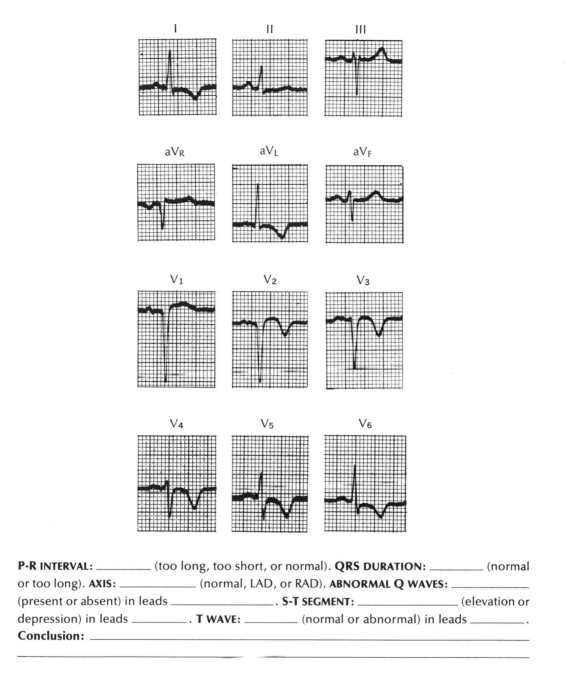

P-R INTERVAL: _____ (too long, too short, or normal). **QRS DURATION:** _____ (normal or too long). **AXIS:** _____ (normal, LAD, or RAD). **ABNORMAL Q WAVES:** _____ (present or absent) in leads _____ . **S-T SEGMENT:** _____ (elevation or depression) in leads _____ . **T WAVE:** _____ (normal or abnormal) in leads _____ .
Conclusion: _____

_____

ANALYSIS

P-R INTERVAL: 0.16 sec. (normal). **QRS DURATION:** 0.08 sec. (normal). **AXIS:** normal. **S-T SEGMENT:** ↑ V_1 and V_2. **T WAVE INVERSION:** I, aV_L, and V_2 to V_6. **ABNORMAL Q WAVES:** aV_L, V_1, and V_2.

Conclusion: This is a subacute (evolving) anteroseptal and lateral wall myocardial infarction. Most of the acute signs of infarction (S-T elevation) have evolved into T wave inversion with a typical arrow shape to the T waves. The S-T segments in the leads reflecting the anterior and lateral walls are typically coved upward.

EXERCISE 9-7

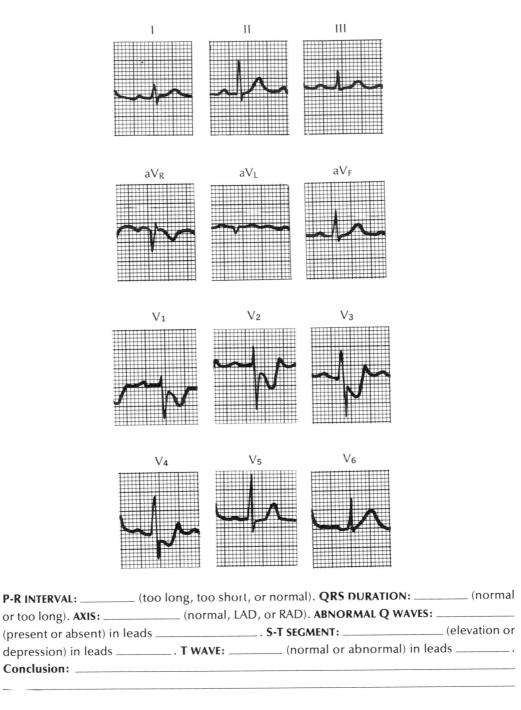

P-R INTERVAL: _____ (too long, too short, or normal). **QRS DURATION:** _____ (normal or too long). **AXIS:** _____ (normal, LAD, or RAD). **ABNORMAL Q WAVES:** _____ (present or absent) in leads _____ . **S-T SEGMENT:** _____ (elevation or depression) in leads _____ . **T WAVE:** _____ (normal or abnormal) in leads _____ .
Conclusion: _____

ANALYSIS

P-R INTERVAL: 0.20 sec. (normal). **QRS DURATION:** 0.08 sec. (normal). **AXIS:** normal. **S-T SEGMENT:** ↓ V_1 to V_4. **T WAVE INVERSION:** absent. **ABNORMAL Q WAVES:** absent.

Conclusion: This is an acute, true posterior myocardial infarction. In this ECG you have the opportunity to see changes that are purely reciprocal. This is because none of the routine twelve leads faces this surface of the heart. However, the leads on the opposite side of the heart will reflect reciprocal changes (anterior leads). That is, instead of abnormal Q waves and S-T elevation, there will be an increase in the height and width of the R waves and S-T depression, especially in leads V_1 and V_2.

EXERCISE 9-8

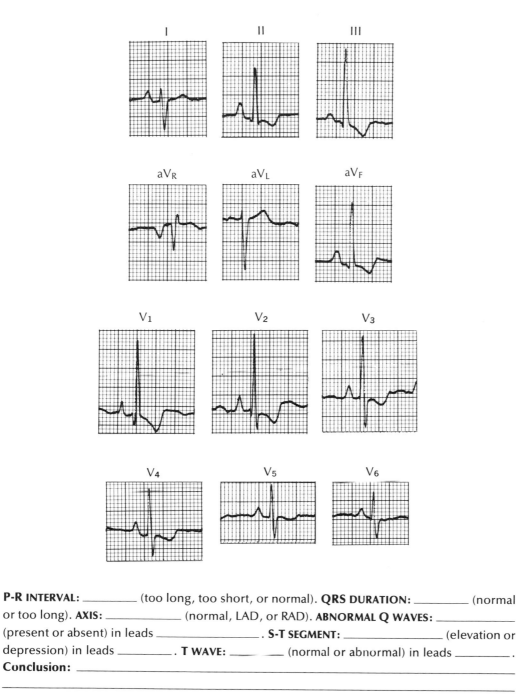

I	II	III
aVR	aVL	aVF
V1	V2	V3
V4	V5	V6

P-R INTERVAL: _____ (too long, too short, or normal). **QRS DURATION:** _____ (normal or too long). **AXIS:** _____ (normal, LAD, or RAD). **ABNORMAL Q WAVES:** _____ (present or absent) in leads _____ . **S-T SEGMENT:** _____ (elevation or depression) in leads _____ . **T WAVE:** _____ (normal or abnormal) in leads _____ .
Conclusion: _____
_____

ANALYSIS

P-R INTERVAL: 0.16 sec. (normal). **QRS DURATION:** 0.10 sec. **AXIS:** RAD. **S-T SEGMENT:** ↓ V_2 to V_5. **T WAVE INVERSION:** V_1 to V_5, II, III, and aV_F. **ABNORMAL Q WAVES:** absent.
Conclusion: This is right ventricular hypertrophy. Because of the prominent R wave in lead V_1, it must be differentiated from true posterior myocardial infarction. When right axis deviation and right atrial enlargement accompany such a morphology in lead V_1, the diagnosis of right ventricular hypertrophy (RVH) is more likely. Minimal QRS prolongation is seen, probably reflective of incomplete RBBB, which is sometimes additional evidence of RVH.

RBBB and LPH will also have a primarily positive deflection in lead V_1 with RAD. However, in RBBB the ventricular activation time will be longer than it is in RVH, since RBBB is a late event, and RVH will manifest itself at the beginning of the QRS complex. More precisely, in RVH the R wave in lead V_1 will peak at 0.03-0.05 sec. In RBBB it will occur at 0.06 sec. or more. In addition, the duration of the QRS complex in RVH will be less than 0.12 sec. In RBBB it will be longer than that.

When it is difficult to make a differential diagnosis, a vectorcardiogram occasionally is helpful.

EXERCISE 9-9

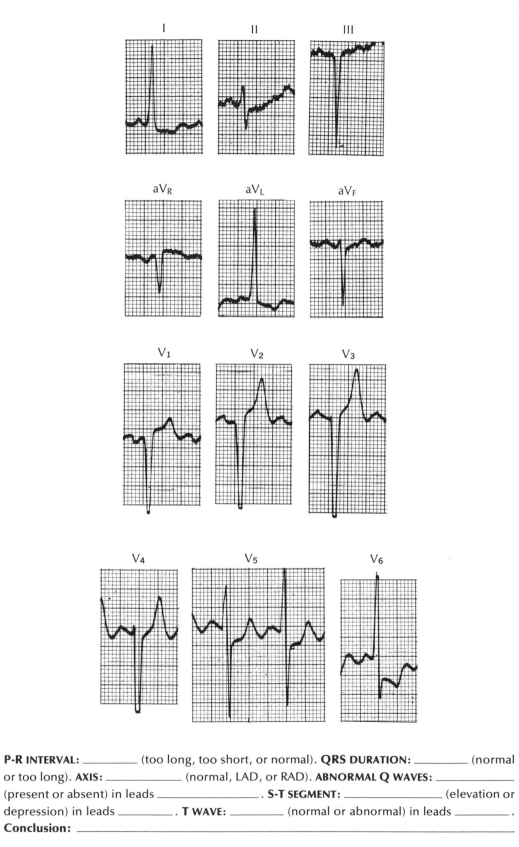

P-R INTERVAL: _____ (too long, too short, or normal). **QRS DURATION:** _____ (normal or too long). **AXIS:** _____ (normal, LAD, or RAD). **ABNORMAL Q WAVES:** _____ (present or absent) in leads _____ . **S-T SEGMENT:** _____ (elevation or depression) in leads _____ . **T WAVE:** _____ (normal or abnormal) in leads _____ .
Conclusion: _____
_____

ANALYSIS

P-R INTERVAL: 0.19 sec. (normal). **QRS DURATION:** 0.09 sec. **AXIS:** LAD. **S-T SEGMENT:** ↑ V_1 to V_3. ↓ I and V_4 to V_6. **T WAVE INVERSION:** V_6 and aV_L. **QS COMPLEXES:** III and V_1 to V_3. **Conclusion:** This ECG represents left ventricular hypertrophy (LVH). It may be confused with myocardial infarction because of poor R wave progression (QS complexes from V_1 to V_3). Anteroseptal myocardial infarction may also be present, however. A vectorcardiogram may be helpful in distinguishing between the two.

EXERCISE 9-10

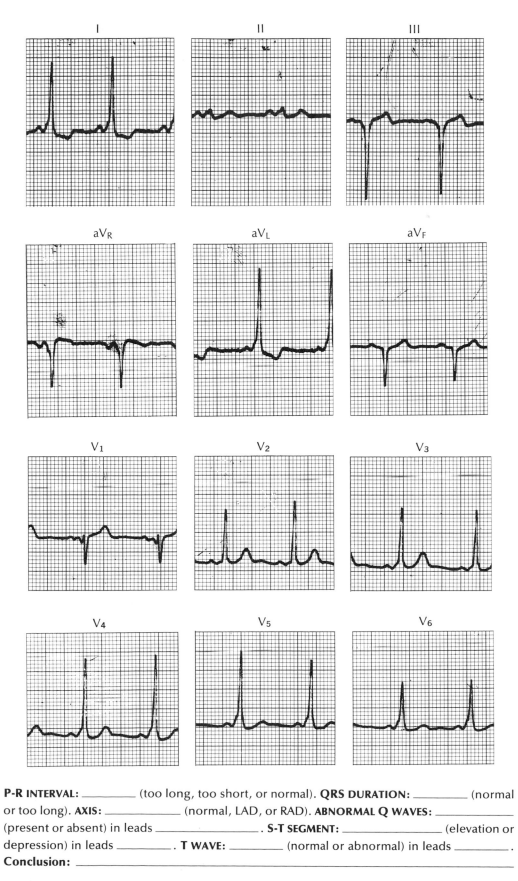

P-R INTERVAL: _____ (too long, too short, or normal). **QRS DURATION:** _____ (normal or too long). **AXIS:** _____ (normal, LAD, or RAD). **ABNORMAL Q WAVES:** _____ (present or absent) in leads _____ . **S-T SEGMENT:** _____ (elevation or depression) in leads _____ . **T WAVE:** _____ (normal or abnormal) in leads _____ .
Conclusion: _____

ANALYSIS

P-R INTERVAL: 0.08 sec. (too short). **QRS DURATION:** 0.12 sec. (too long). **AXIS:** normal. **S-T SEGMENT:** normal. **T WAVE INVERSION:** none. **ABNORMAL Q WAVES:** III, aV$_F$, and V$_1$.

Conclusion: This is Wolff-Parkinson-White (WPW) syndrome, type B. It must be differentiated from inferior wall myocardial infarction because of the pathological Q waves that sometimes appear in the inferior leads. These Q waves are really the result of the slurred initial component of the QRS complex, known as a delta wave.

Delta waves can be seen in this ECG in all leads. Other signs of Wolff-Parkinson-White syndrome are the short P-R interval and long QRS duration.

EXERCISE 9-11

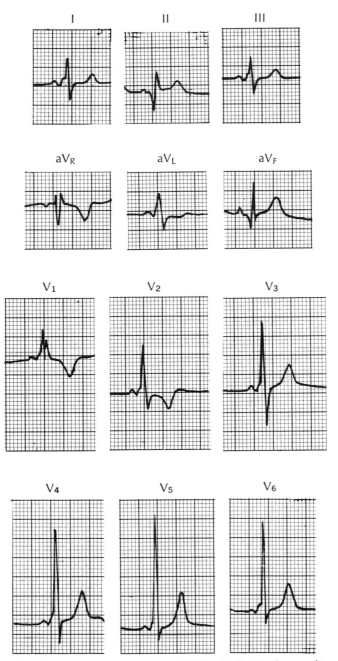

I   II   III

aV_R   aV_L   aV_F

V₁   V₂   V₃

V₄   V₅   V₆

Modified from Conover, M. H., and Zalis, E. G.: Understanding electrocardiography, ed. 2, St. Louis, 1976, The C. V. Mosby Co.

ANALYSIS

P-R INTERVAL: 0.09 sec. (too short). **QRS DURATION:** 0.12 sec. (too long). **AXIS:** normal. **S-T SEGMENT:** normal. **T WAVE INVERSION:** none. **ABNORMAL Q WAVES:** III and aV_F.
Conclusion: Here again is a Wolff-Parkinson-White syndrome. The positive QRS in lead V₁ indicates a type A. The presence of all of the classical signs of preexcitation (short P-R, long QRS, and delta waves) would differentiate this tracing from inferior wall myocardial infarction. The differentiation is necessary because of the abnormal Q waves (delta forces) in leads II and aV_F.

235

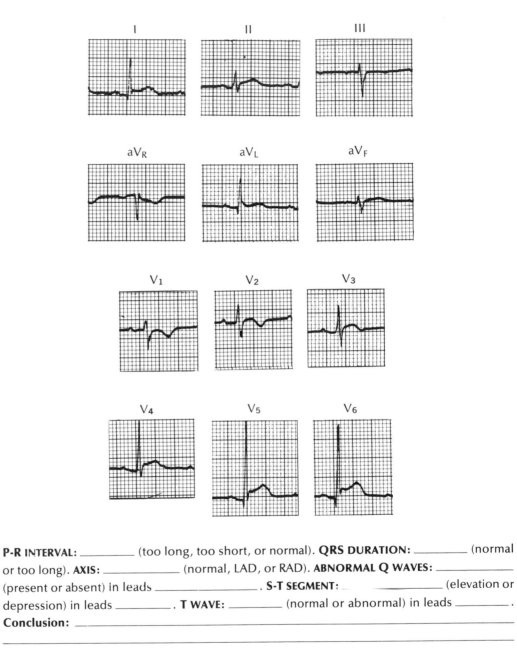

P-R INTERVAL: _____ (too long, too short, or normal). **QRS DURATION:** _____ (normal or too long). **AXIS:** _____ (normal, LAD, or RAD). **ABNORMAL Q WAVES:** _____ (present or absent) in leads _____ . **S-T SEGMENT:** _____ (elevation or depression) in leads _____ . **T WAVE:** _____ (normal or abnormal) in leads _____ .
Conclusion: _____

ANALYSIS

P-R INTERVAL: 0.16 sec. (normal). **QRS DURATION:** 0.08 sec. (normal). **AXIS:** normal. **S-T SEGMENT:** ↑ I; ↓ II, aV$_L$, and V$_3$ to V$_6$. **T WAVE INVERSION:** III, V$_1$, and V$_2$. **ABNORMAL Q WAVES:** none.

Conclusion: This tracing represents an acute pericarditis. It must be differentiated from acute myocardial infarction because of the elevated S-T segments seen in the limb leads and left precordial leads and because of T wave inversion.

In acute pericarditis the S-T segment elevation is not accompanied by reciprocal S-T depression. For example, in the above tracing there is S-T elevation in both leads I and III. The shape of the S-T segment in pericarditis is typically concave upward instead of convex, as in myocardial infarction. The ECG of pericarditis evolves quickly, within a few weeks, and *Q waves will not appear.*

Characteristically the S-T segments in acute pericarditis will be elevated in many leads with upright T waves except in lead III, which may be inverted. After this the S-T segment becomes isoelectric, and there is widespread T wave inversion. The S-T and T wave changes take place in the course of several weeks.

EXERCISE 9-13

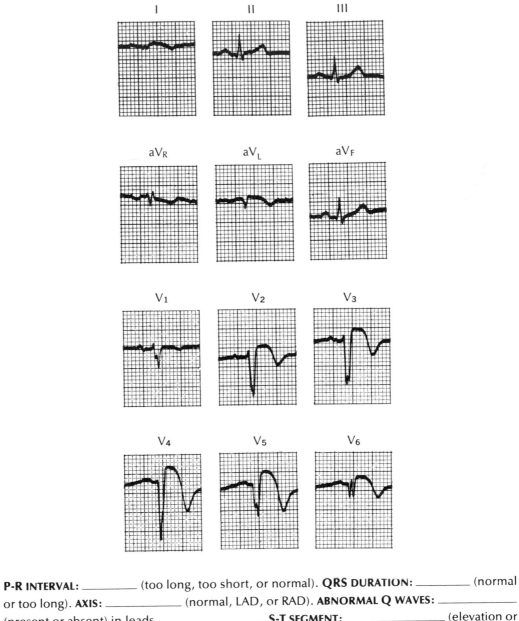

P-R INTERVAL: _____ (too long, too short, or normal). **QRS DURATION:** _____ (normal or too long). **AXIS:** _____ (normal, LAD, or RAD). **ABNORMAL Q WAVES:** _____ (present or absent) in leads _____ . **S-T SEGMENT:** _____ (elevation or depression) in leads _____ . **T WAVE:** _____ (normal or abnormal) in leads _____ .

Conclusion: _____

ANALYSIS

P-R INTERVAL: 0.16 sec. (normal). **QRS DURATION:** 0.09 sec. **AXIS:** normal. **S-T SEGMENT:** ↑ V_2 to V_6. **T WAVE INVERSION:** I, aV_L, and V_1 to V_6. **ABNORMAL Q WAVES:** I, aV_L, V_5, and V_6.

Conclusion: This ECG reflects an acute, anteroseptal myocardial infarction with extension to the lateral wall.

CHAPTER 10
TEST TRACINGS

This chapter should give you a fair idea of what you need to study and where your weaknesses are. There are sixty tracings, all taken from examinations I have given in the past. The background needed to give correct answers to the first forty tracings is what is generally considered basic knowledge and a prerequisite for coronary care nursing. Mixed in with the remainder of the tracings are rhythms reflecting less apparent mechanisms, but all are within the grasp of the experienced coronary care nurse. Answers appear at the end of the chapter.

Remember to look for first-degree heart block by measuring the P-R intervals, intraventricular conduction anomalies by measuring the QRS duration, and a regular rhythm versus premature beats by walking out the P waves and R waves.

Other things to remember are:
1. The most common cause of an unexpected pause is a nonconducted PAC.
2. The abrupt onset of an apparent sinus bradycardia may really be bigeminal nonconducted PACs.
3. Atrial fibrillation treated with digitalis should still have an absolutely irregular ventricular response and an adequate rate.
4. Second-degree heart block with 2:1 conduction can be either type I or type II. You cannot know which type unless there are two conducted beats in a row.
5. Whenever you make a diagnosis of second-degree block with a 2:1 conduction ratio, be absolutely sure that the P-R intervals are all the same. You may be dealing with complete heart block.
6. A full compensatory pause is *not* conclusive of ventricular ectopy. It is conclusive of nothing. When it is *less than full*, it indicates premature atrial activity.

EXERCISE 10-1

II

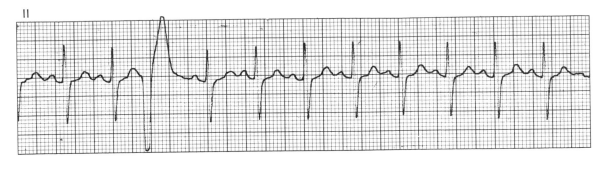

Conclusion: _____

_____

EXERCISE 10-2

V₁

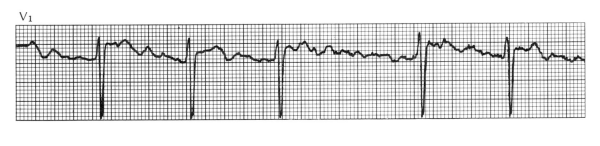

Conclusion: _____

_____

EXERCISE 10-3

II

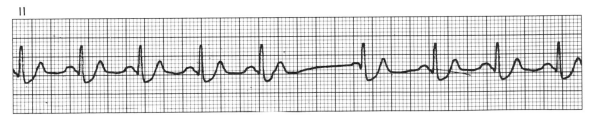

Conclusion: _____

_____

EXERCISE 10-4

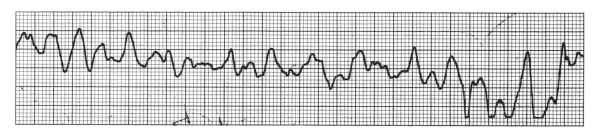

Conclusion: _____

_____

EXERCISE 10-5

II

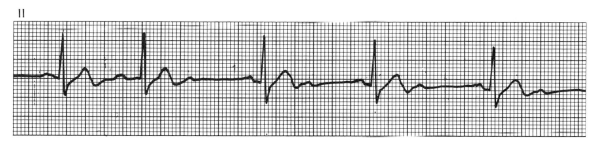

Conclusion: _____

_____

EXERCISE 10-6

II

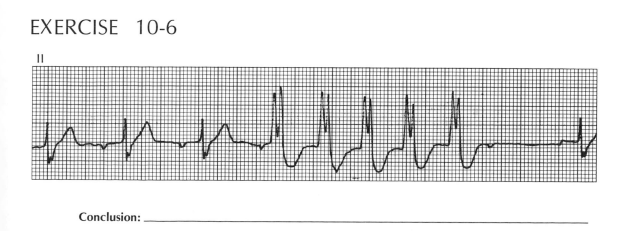

Conclusion: _____

_____

EXERCISE 10-7

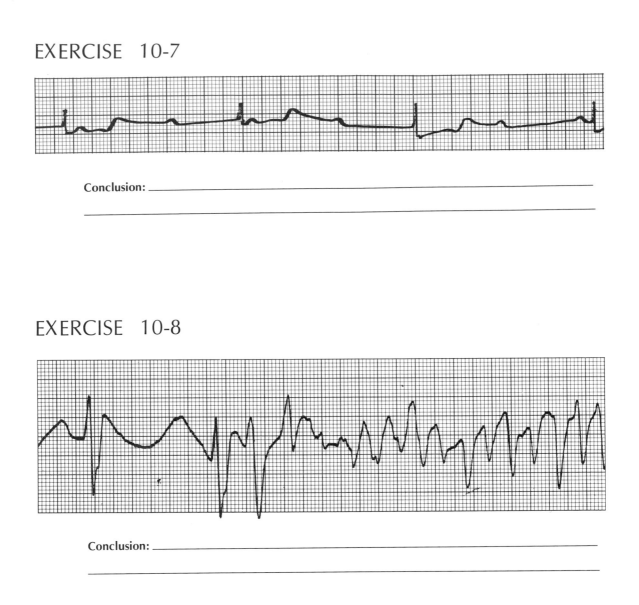

Conclusion: _____

_____

EXERCISE 10-8

Conclusion: _____

_____

EXERCISE 10-9

II

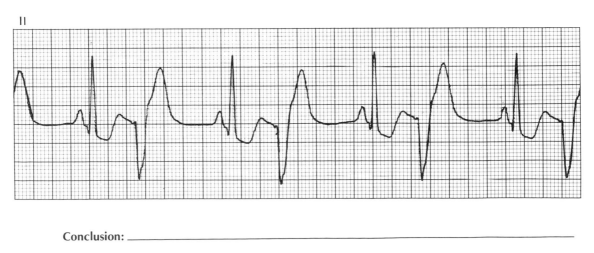

Conclusion: _____

_____

EXERCISE 10-10

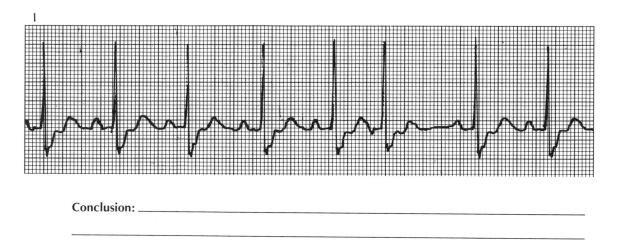

Conclusion: _____

_____

EXERCISE 10-11

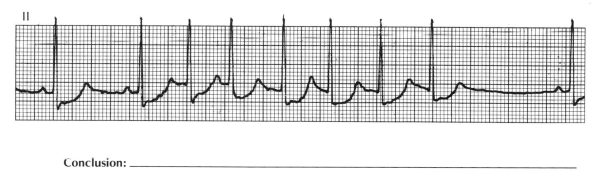

Conclusion: _____

_____

EXERCISE 10-12

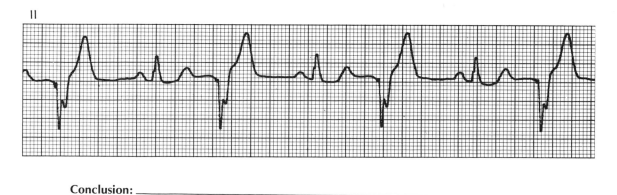

Conclusion: _____

_____

EXERCISE 10-13

II

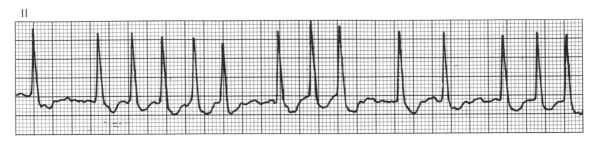

Conclusion: _____

_____

EXERCISE 10-14

V₁

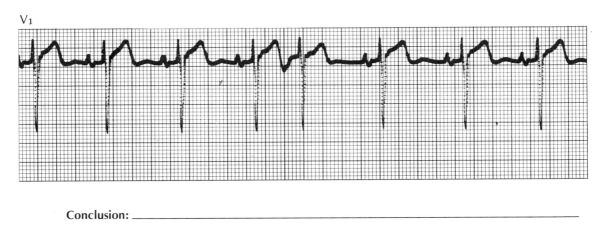

Conclusion: _____

_____

EXERCISE 10-15

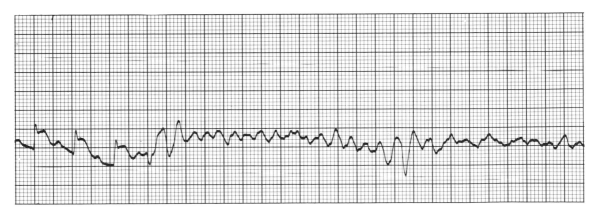

Conclusion: _____

_____

EXERCISE 10-16

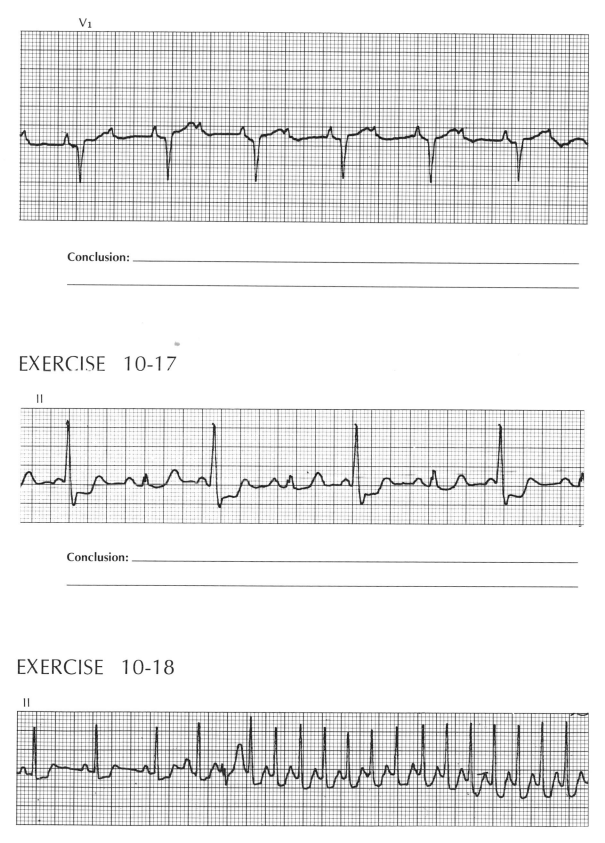

V_1

Conclusion: _____

_____

EXERCISE 10-17

II

Conclusion: _____

_____

EXERCISE 10-18

II

Conclusion: _____

_____

EXERCISE 10-19

V₁

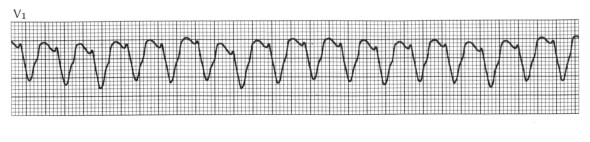

Conclusion: _____

_____

EXERCISE 10-20

II

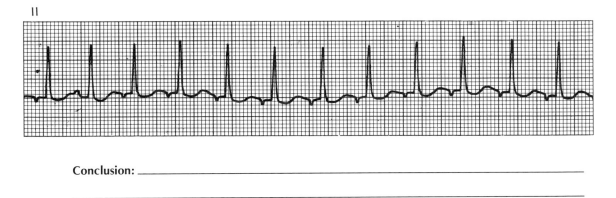

Conclusion: _____

_____

EXERCISE 10-21

V₁

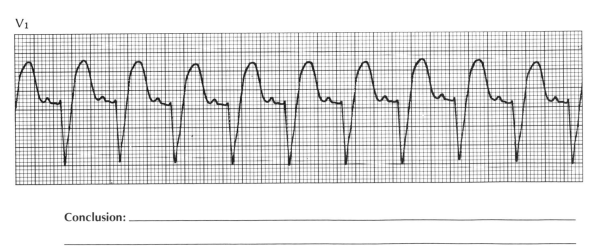

Conclusion: _____

_____

246

EXERCISE 10-22

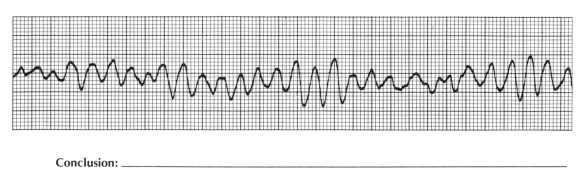

Conclusion: _____

_____

EXERCISE 10-23

V₁

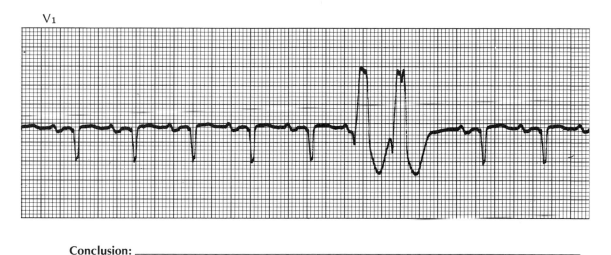

Conclusion: _____

_____

EXERCISE 10-24

V₁

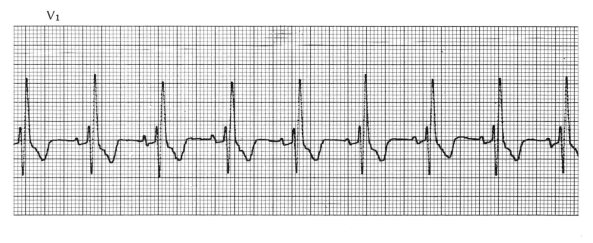

Conclusion: _____

_____

EXERCISE 10-25

II

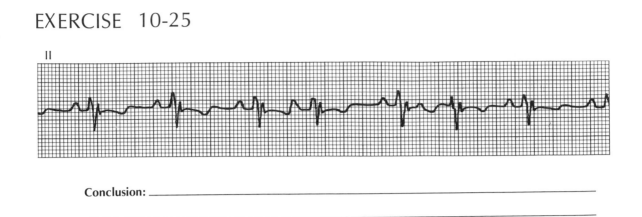

Conclusion: _____

_____

EXERCISE 10-26

III

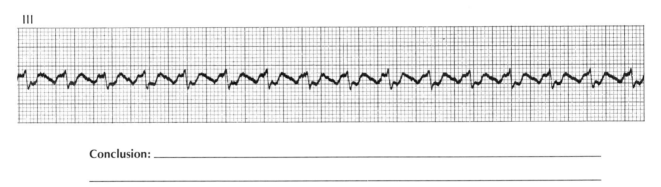

Conclusion: _____

_____

EXERCISE 10-27

V₁

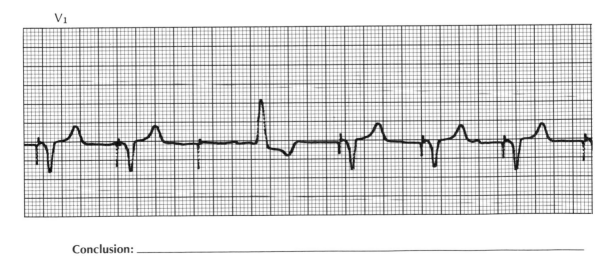

Conclusion: _____

_____

EXERCISE 10-28

II

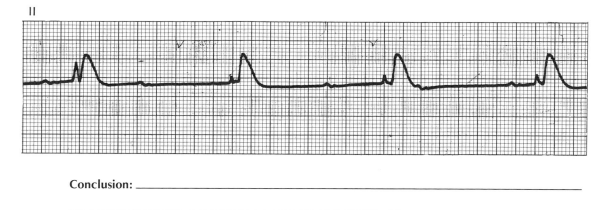

Conclusion: _____

_____

EXERCISE 10-29

II

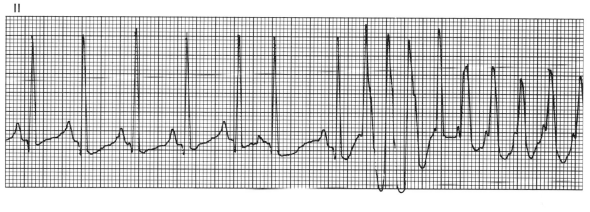

Conclusion: _____

_____

EXERCISE 10-30

V$_1$

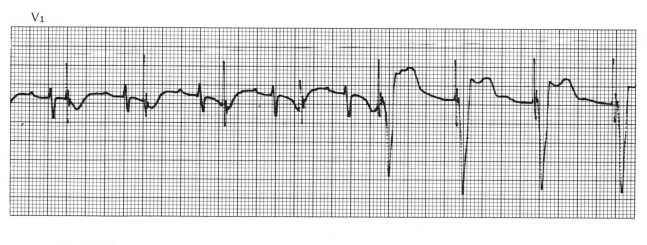

Conclusion: _____

_____

EXERCISE 10-31

V₁

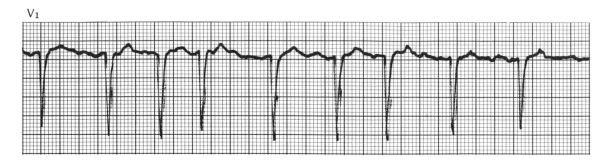

Conclusion: _____

_____

EXERCISE 10-32

II

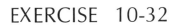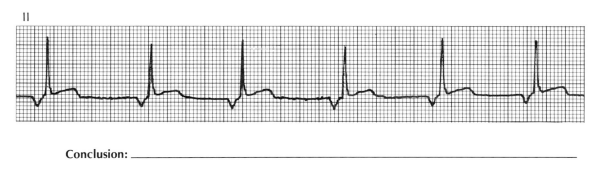

Conclusion: _____

_____

EXERCISE 10-33

II

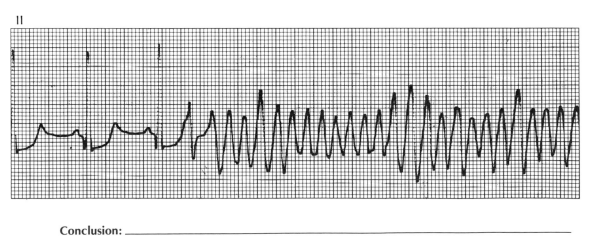

Conclusion: _____

_____

EXERCISE 10-34

II

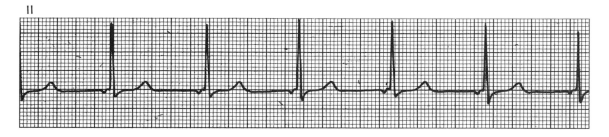

Conclusion: _____

_____

EXERCISE 10-35

II

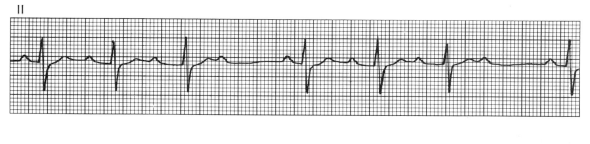

Conclusion: _____

_____

EXERCISE 10-36

II

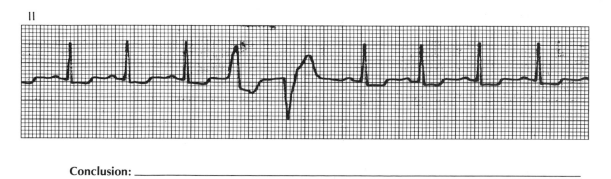

Conclusion: _____

_____

EXERCISE 10-37

V₁

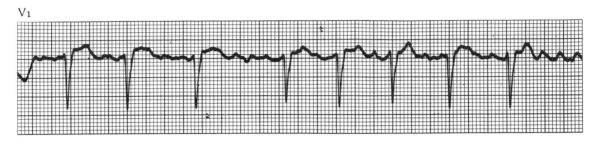

Conclusion: _____

_____

EXERCISE 10-38

II

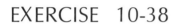
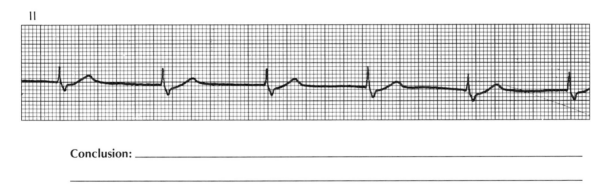

Conclusion: _____

_____

EXERCISE 10-39

II

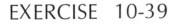
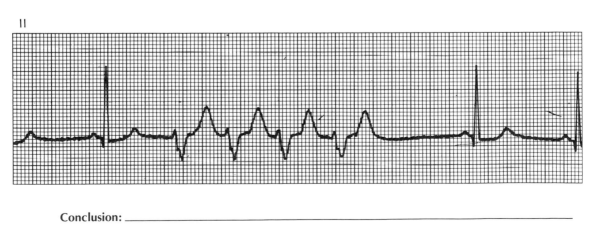

Conclusion: _____

_____

EXERCISE 10-40

II

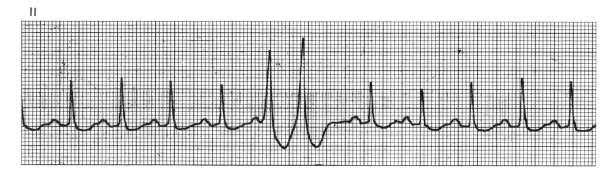

Conclusion: _____

_____

EXERCISE 10-41

V₁

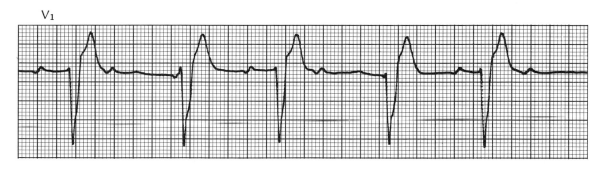

Conclusion: _____

_____

EXERCISE 10-42

II

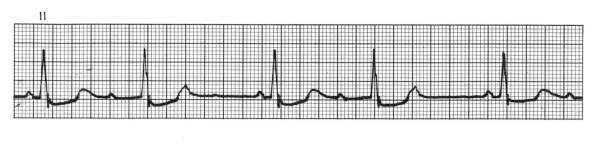

Conclusion: _____

_____

EXERCISE 10-43

V₁

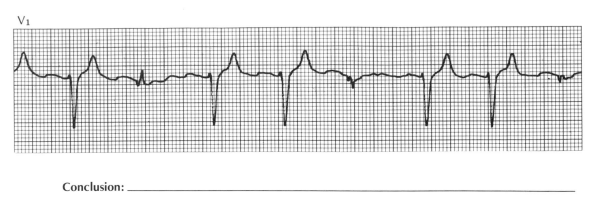

Conclusion: _____

_____

EXERCISE 10-44

II

Conclusion: _____

_____

EXERCISE 10-45

II

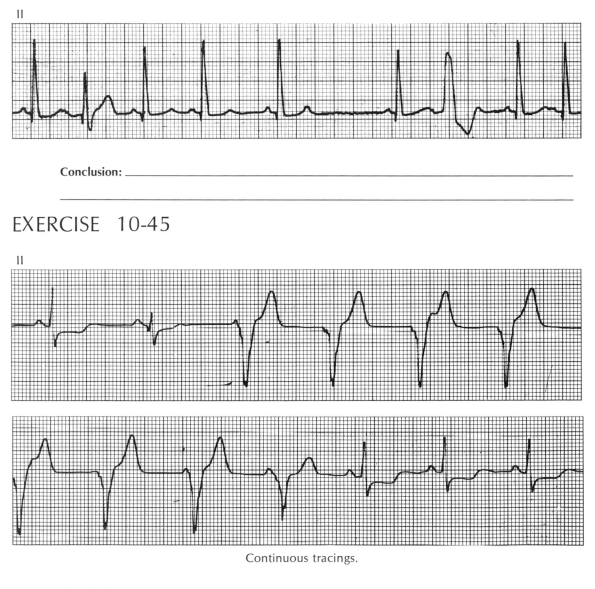

Continuous tracings.

Conclusion: _____

_____

EXERCISE   10-46

II

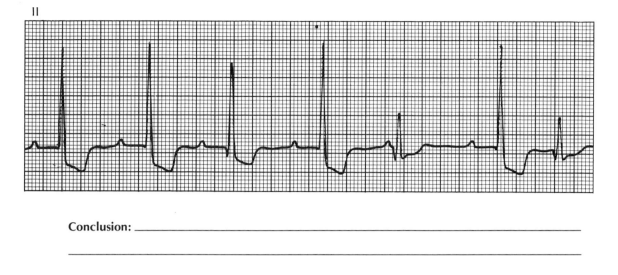

Conclusion: _____

_____

EXERCISE   10-47

II

Conclusion: _____

_____

EXERCISE   10-48

II

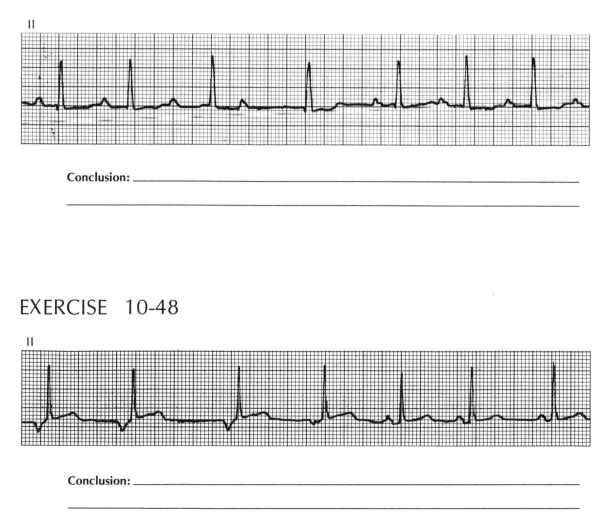

Conclusion: _____

_____

EXERCISE 10-49

II

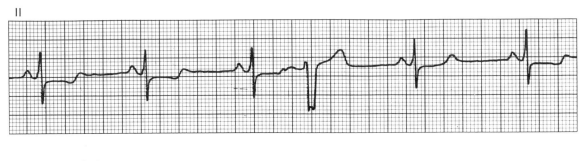

Conclusion: _____

_____

EXERCISE 10-50

II

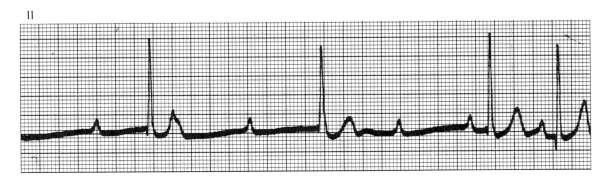

Conclusion: _____

_____

EXERCISE 10-51

V₁

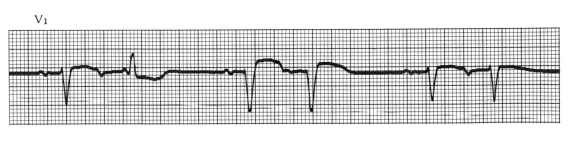

Conclusion: _____

_____

EXERCISE 10-52

V₁

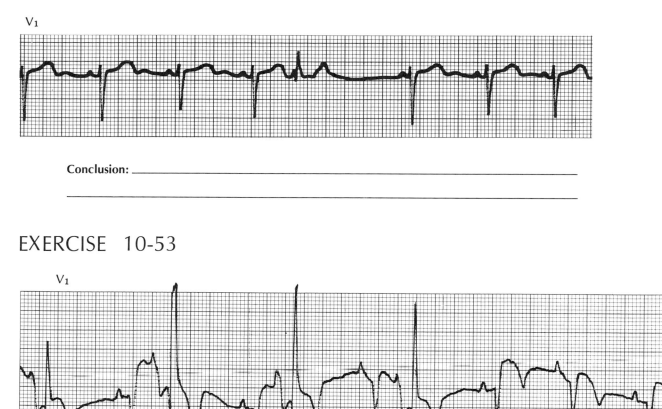

Conclusion: _____

_____

EXERCISE 10-53

V₁

Conclusion: _____

_____

EXERCISE 10-54

II

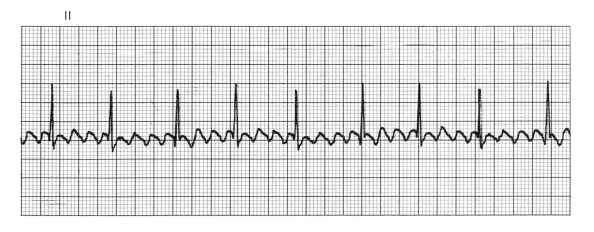

Conclusion: _____

_____

EXERCISE 10-55

V₁

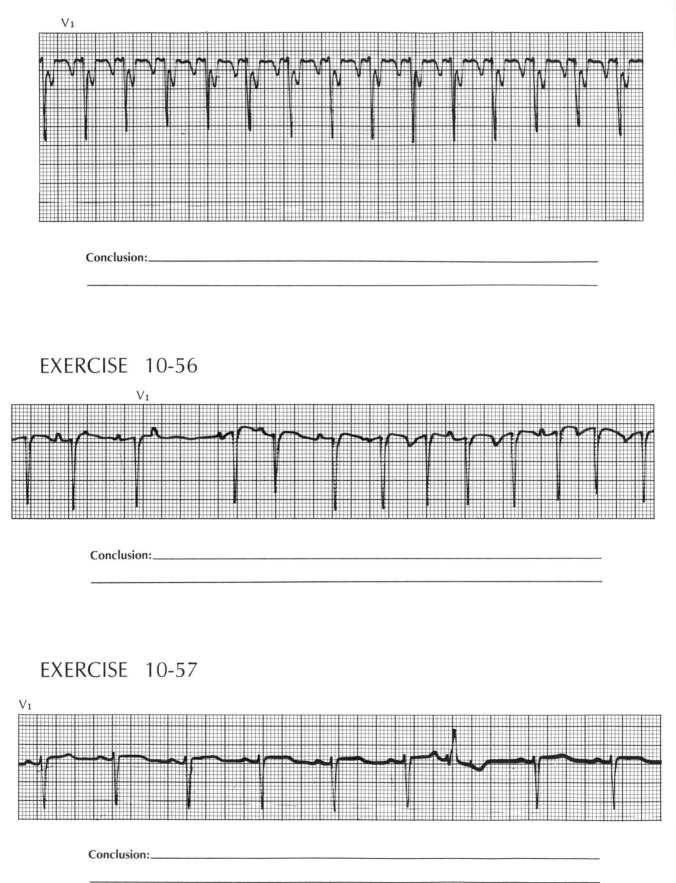

Conclusion:_____

_____

EXERCISE 10-56

V₁

Conclusion:_____

_____

EXERCISE 10-57

V₁

Conclusion:_____

_____

EXERCISE 10-58

II

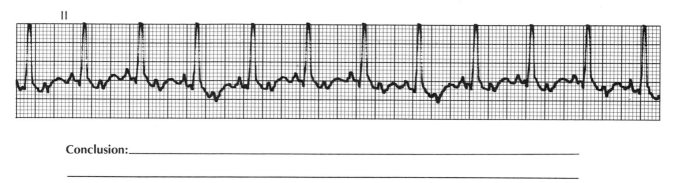

Conclusion:_____

_____

EXERCISE 10-59

V₁

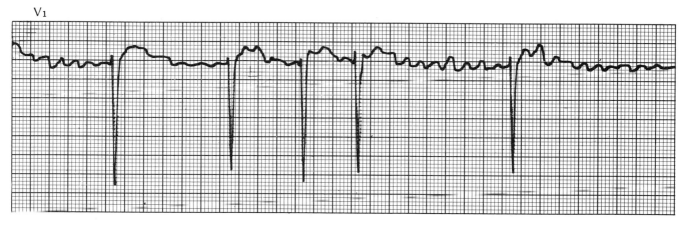

Conclusion:_____

_____

EXERCISE 10-60

II

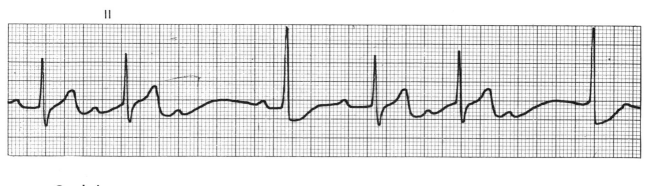

Conclusion:_____

_____

ANSWERS

10-1	Sinus tachycardia with one PVC.
10-2	Atrial fibrillation with too much A-V block, perhaps digitalis excess.
10-3	Normal sinus rhythm with a nonconducted PAC, followed by a junctional escape beat.
10-4	Ventricular fibrillation.
10-5	Type I (Wenckebach 3:2 and 2:1) second-degree A-V block.
10-6	First-degree heart block and paroxysmal ventricular tachycardia.
10-7	Complete heart block.
10-8	Paired PVCs, resulting in ventricular fibrillation.
10-9	Bigeminal ventricular ectopics.
10-10	Normal sinus rhythm with one PAC and probably underlying BBB (R).
10-11	Paroxysmal supraventricular tachycardia.
10-12	Bigeminal ventricular ectopics.
10-13	Atrial fibrillation.
10-14	Normal sinus rhythm with a PAC.
10-15	Paired end-diastolic PVCs resulting in ventricular fibrillation.
10-16	Atrial tachycardia (130/min.) with 2:1 A-V conduction.
10-17	Bigeminal end-diastolic PVCs.
10-18	Paroxysmal supraventricular tachycardia.
10-19	Ventricular tachycardia.
10-20	Nonparoxysmal junctional tachycardia.
10-21	Sinus tachycardia with LBBB.
10-22	Ventricular fibrillation.
10-23	First-degree heart block and paired end-diastolic PVCs.
10-24	Normal sinus rhythm with RBBB.
10-25	Normal sinus rhythm with two PACs.
10-26	Atrial flutter with 2:1 A-V conduction.
10-27	Pacemaker rhythm with one noncapture. Patient's own rhythm reflects first-degree heart block and RBBB.
10-28	Complete heart block.
10-29	Sinus tachycardia, PAC (sixth P wave), and R-on-T phenomenon triggering ventricular tachycardia.
10-30	Malfunctioning demand pacemaker or fixed rate competing with patient's own rhythm, firing on the T wave. Last half of the strip shows capture.
10-31	Atrial fibrillation.
10-32	Escape junctional rhythm.
10-33	R-on-T phenomenon resulting in ventricular fibrillation.
10-34	Junctional rhythm, escape (60/min.).
10-35	Type I (Wenckebach 4:3) second-degree heart block.
10-36	Multiform paired PVCs.
10-37	Atrial fibrillation.
10-38	Escape junctional rhythm.
10-39	Sinus bradycardia with paroxysmal ventricular tachycardia.
10-40	Sinus tachycardia with paired end-diastolic PVCs.
10-41	Second-degree heart block with 2:1 A-V conduction, junctional escape beats, and an underlying LBBB.
10-42	Type I (Wenckebach 3:2) second-degree heart block.
10-43	Trigeminal end-diastolic PVCs, all of which are fusion beats.
10-44	There are five PACs occurring every other beat. Two of them are con-

ducted with aberration, and one is not conducted at all. A junctional escape beat follows the pause.

10-45 Accelerated idioventricular rhythm, beginning and ending with fusion beats.

10-46 Ventricular parasystole and first-degree heart block. Note no fixed coupling and one fusion beat (third complex).

10-47 Type I (Wenckebach 4:3) second-degree heart block with one junctional escape beat (fourth complex).

10-48 Wandering pacemaker with one atrial fusion beat (fourth P wave). There is an underlying sinus arrhythmia.

10-49 Sinus bradycardia with one PAC aberrantly conducted.

10-50 Intermittent complete heart block.

10-51 Bigeminal PACs. The first one is conducted with RBBB aberration.

10-52 Sinus arrhythmia with a prominent U wave and one PAC conducted with RBBB aberration.

10-53 Bigeminal PACs conducted with RBBB aberration.

10-54 Atrial flutter with 4:1 A-V conduction.

10-55 Atrial flutter with 2:1 A-V conduction.

10-56 Chaotic atrial tachycardia with one nonconducted PAC.

10-57 Normal sinus rhythm with one PAC conducted with RBBB aberration.

10-58 Atrial tachycardia (200/min.) with a 2:1 A-V conduction ratio.

10-59 Atrial fibrillation and profound bradycardia, perhaps from digitalis excess.

10-60 Type I (Wenckebach 3:2) second-degree heart block with junctional escape beats (third and last complexes).

APPENDIX

NORMAL Q-T INTERVALS AND THE UPPER LIMITS OF THE NORMAL*

Heart rate per minute	Men and children (sec.)	Women (sec.)	Upper limits of the normal	
			Men and children (sec.)	Women (sec.)
40.0	0.449	0.461	0.491	0.503
43.0	0.438	0.450	0.479	0.491
46.0	0.426	0.438	0.466	0.478
48.0	0.420	0.432	0.460	0.471
50.0	0.414	0.425	0.453	0.464
52.0	0.407	0.418	0.445	0.456
54.5	0.400	0.411	0.438	0.449
57.0	0.393	0.404	0.430	0.441
60.0	0.386	0.396	0.422	0.432
63.0	0.378	0.388	0.413	0.423
66.5	0.370	0.380	0.404	0.414
70.5	0.361	0.371	0.395	0.405
75.0	0.352	0.362	0.384	0.394
80.0	0.342	0.352	0.374	0.384
86.0	0.332	0.341	0.363	0.372
92.5	0.321	0.330	0.351	0.360
100.0	0.310	0.318	0.338	0.347
109.0	0.297	0.305	0.325	0.333
120.0	0.283	0.291	0.310	0.317
133.0	0.268	0.276	0.294	0.301
150.0	0.252	0.258	0.275	0.282
172.0	0.234	0.240	0.255	0.262

*From Ashman, R., and Hull, E.: Essentials of electrocardiography, New York, 1945, Macmillan, Inc.; reproduced with the kind permission of Edgar Hull, M.D.

REFERENCES

GENERAL

1. Conover, M. H., and Zalis, E. G.: Understanding electrocardiography, ed. 2, St. Louis, 1976, The C. V. Mosby Co.
2. Hurst, J. W., editor: The heart, ed. 3, New York, 1974, McGraw-Hill Book Co.
3. Marriott, H. J. L.: Practical electrocardiography, ed. 5, Baltimore, 1972, The Williams & Wilkins Co.
4. Pribble, A., and Preston, T. A.: Electrocardiographic changes. In Zschoche, D. A.: Mosby's comprehensive review of critical care, St. Louis, 1976, The C. V. Mosby Co.

SICK SINUS SYNDROME

5. Easley, R. M., and Goldstein, S.: Sinoatrial syncope, Am. J. Med. **50:**166, 1971.
6. Eraul, D., and Shaw, D. B.: Sinus bradycardia, Br. Heart J. **33:**742, 1971.
7. Ferrer, M. I.: The sick sinus syndrome in atrial disease, J.A.M.A. **206:**645, 1968.
8. Ferrer, M. I.: The sick sinus syndrome, Circulation **47:**635, 1973.
9. Freulian, C. T., Obeid, A. L., Smulyan, H., and others: Sick sinus syndrome; one year's experience (abstract), Circulation **41-42**(suppl. 3):154, 1970.
10. Kaplan, B. M., Langendorf, R., Lev, M., and Pick, A.: Tachycardia-bradycardia syndrome (so-called "sick sinus syndrome"); pathology, mechanisms, and treatment, Am. J. Cardiol. **31:**497, 1973.
11. Rosen, K. M., Loeb, H. S., Sinno, M. Z., and others: Cardiac conduction in patients with symptomatic sinus node disease, Circulation **43:**836, 1971.
12. Rubenstein, J. J., Schulman, C. L., Yurchak, P. M., and other: Clinical spectrum of the sick sinus syndrome, Circulation, **46:**5, 1972.
13. Schulman, C. L., Rubenstein, J. J., Yurchak, P. M., and others: The "sick sinus" syndrome; clinical spectrum (abstract), Circulation **41-42** (suppl. 3):42, 1970.
14. Sigurd, B., Jensen, G., Melbon, J., and others: Adams-Stokes syndrome caused by sinoatrial block, Br. Heart J. **35:**1002, 1973.

SINUS NODE DEPRESSION BY ATRIAL ECTOPY (OVERDRIVE SUPPRESSION)

15. Lange, G.: Action of driving stimuli from intrinsic and extrinsic sources on in situ cardiac pacemaker tissues, Circ. Res. **17:**449, 1965.
16. Mandel, W., Hayakawa, H., Danzig, R., and others: Evaluation of sino-atrial node function in man by overdrive suppression, Circulation **44:**59, 1971.
17. Meisner, M. H., Rich, J. M., Fontana, M. E., and others: Sinoatrial recovery time in man (abstract), Circulation **41-42**(suppl. 3):183, 1970.
18. Narula, O. S., Samet, P., and Javier, R. P.: Significance of the sinus node recovery time, Circulation **45:**140, 1972.
19. Pick, A., Langendorf, R., and Katz, L. N.: Depression of cardiac pacemakers by premature impulses, Am. Heart J. **41:**49, 1951.

ARRHYTHMIAS AND CORONARY BLOOD FLOW

20. Benchimol, A., Matsuo, S., and others: Phasic coronary arterial flow velocity during arrhythmias in man, Am. J. Cardiol. **29:**604, 1972.
21. Corday, E., Gold, H., and others: Effect of the cardiac arrhythmias on the coronary circulation, Ann. Intern. Med. **50:**535, 1959.
22. Pitt, B., and Gregg, D. E.: Coronary hemodynamic effects of increasing ventricular rate in the unanesthetized dog, Circ. Res. **22:**753, 1968.
23. Wegria, R., Frank, C. W., Wang, H. H., and others: The effect of atrial and ventricular tachycardia on cardiac output, coronary blood flow, and mean arterial blood pressure, Circ. Res. **6:**624, 1958.

SINUS BRADYCARDIA AND THE USE OF ATROPINE

24. Beisner, G. D., Rosing, D. R., and others: Treatment of ventricular arrhythmias occurring during acute coronary artery occlusion in conscious dogs, Am. J. Cardiol. **29:**253, 1972.
25. Braunwald, E., Covell, J. W., Maroko, P. R., and Ross, J., Jr.: Effects of drugs and of counterpulsation on myocardial oxygen consumption; observations on the ischemic heart, Circulation **41**(suppl. 4):220, 1969.
26. Chadda, K. D., Banka, V. S., and Helfant, R. H.: Rate dependent ventricular ectopia following acute coronary occlusion; the concept of an optimal antiarrhythmic heart rate, Circulation **49:**654, 1974.
27. Epstein, S. E., Redwood, D. R., and Smith, E. R.: Atropine and acute myocardial infarction, Circulation **47:**430, 1973.
28. Goldstein, R. E., Darsh, R. B., Smith, E. R., and others: Influence of atropine and of vagally mediated bradycardia on the occurrence of ventricular arrhythmias following acute coronary occlusion in closed-chest dogs, Circulation **47:**1180, 1973.
29. Han, J.: Atropine and acute myocardial infarction, Circulation **47:**429, 1973.
30. Karish, R. B., Orlando, M., and others: Ineffectiveness of prophylactic atropine in decreasing arrhythmias and enhancing survival following acute coronary artery occlusion in conscious dogs, Am. J. Cardiol. **29:**273, 1972.
31. Kent, K. M., Smith, E. R., and others: The deleterious electrophysiological effects produced by increasing heart rate during experimental coronary occlusion, Circ. Res. **20:**379, 1972.

32. Maroko, P. R., Kjekshus, J. K., and others: Factors influencing infarct size following experimental coronary artery occlusion, Circulation **43**:67, 1971.

33. Massumi, R. A., Mason, D. T., Amsterdam, E. A., and others: Ventricular fibrillation and tachycardia after intravenous atropine for treatment of bradycardias, N. Engl. J. Med. **287**:336, 1972.

34. Myers, R. W., Pearlman, A. S., and others: Beneficial effects of vagal stimulation and bradycardia during experimental acute myocardial ischemia, Circulation **49**:943, 1974.

35. Redwood, D. R., Smith, E. R., and Epstein, S. E.: Coronary artery occlusion in the conscious dogs; effects of alterations in heart rates and arterial pressure on the degree of myocardial ischemia, Circulation **56**:323, 1972.

36. Richman, S.: Adverse effect of atropine during myocardial infarction; enhancement of ischemia following intravenously administered atropine, J.A.M.A. **228**:1414, 1974.

37. Scheinman, M. M., Thorburn, D., and Abbott, J. A.: Use of atropine in patients with acute myocardial infarction and sinus bradycardia, Circulation **52**:627, 1975.

38. Stock, E.: Cardiac slowing not cardiac irritability; the major problem in the prehospital phase of myocardial infarction (abstract), Aust. N.Z. J. Med. **44**:124, 1971.

39. Thomas, M., and Woodgate, D.: Effect of atropine on bradycardia and hypotension in acute myocardial infarction, Br. Heart J. **28**:409, 1966.

CONCEALED JUNCTIONAL ECTOPICS SIMULATING FIRST- AND SECOND-DEGREE HEART BLOCK

40. Castellanos, A., Befeler, B., and Myerburg, R. J.: Psuedo A-V block produced by concealed extrasystoles arising below the bifurcation of the His bundle, Br. Heart J. **36**:457, 1974.

41. Damato, A. M., Lau, S. H., and Bobb, G. A.: Cardiac arrhythmias simulated by concealed bundle of His extrasystoles in the dog, Circ. Res. **28**:316, 1971.

42. El-Sherif, N., Befeler, B., and others: Re-entry due to manifest and concealed His bundle ectopic systoles; report of a case, Circulation **53**:902, 1976.

43. Eugster, G. S., Godfrey, C. C., Brammell, H. L., and Pryor, R.: Psuedo A-V block associated with A-H and H-V conduction defects, Am. Heart J. **85**:789, 1973.

44. Langendorf, R.: Alternation of A-V conduction time, Am. Heart J. **55**:181, 1958.

45. Langendorf, R., and Mehlman, F. S.: Blocked (nonconducted) A-V nodal premature systoles initiating first and second degree A-V block, Am. Heart J. **34**:500, 1947.

46. Langendorf, R., and Pick, A.: Concealed conduction in the A-V junction. In Dreifus, L. S., Likoff, W., and Moyer, J. H., editors: Mechanisms and therapy of cardiac arrhythmias, New York, 1966, Grune & Stratton, Inc.

47. Narula, O. S.: Current concepts of atrioventricular block. In Narula, O. S., editor: His

bundle electrocardiography and clinical electrophysiology, Philadelphia, 1975, F. A. Davis Co.

48. Rosen, K. M., Rahimtoola, S. H., and Gunnar, R. M.: Pseudo A-V block secondary to premature non-propagated His bundle depolarization; documentation by His bundle electrocardiography, Circulation **42**:367, 1970.

A-V NODAL REENTRY

49. Bigger, J. T., Jr., and Goldreter, B. N.: The mechanism of paroxysmal supraventricular tachycardia in man, Circulation **42**:643, 1970.

50. Goldreyer, B. N., and Bigger, J. T. Jr.: The site of reentry in paroxysmal supraventricular tachycardia in man, Circulation **43**:15, 1971.

51. Josephson, M. E., and Kastor, J. A.: Paroxysmal supraventricular tachycardia; is the atrium a necessary link? Circulation **54**:430, 1976.

52. Wellens, H. J. J., Duren, D. R., and others: Effect of digitalis in patients with paroxysmal atrioventricular nodal tachycardia, Circulation **52**:779, 1975.

53. Wellens, H. J. J., Wesdorp, J. C., and others: Second degree block during reciprocal atrioventricular nodal tachycardia, Circulation **53**:595, 1976.

54. Wu, D., Denes, P., and others: Demonstration of dual atrioventricular nodal pathways utilizing a ventricular extrastimulus in patients with atrioventricular nodal re-entrant paroxysmal supraventricular tachycardia, Circulation **52**:789, 1975.

SINUS-NODAL REENTRY AS A CAUSE OF PAROXYSMAL SUPRAVENTRICULAR TACHYCARDIA

55. Bonke, F. I. M., Bouman, L. N., and Schopman, F. J. G.: Effect of an early atrial premature beat on activity of the sino-atrial node and atrial rhythm in the rabbit, Circ. Res. **29**:704, 1971.

56. Childers, R. W., Arnsdorf, M. F., and others: Sinus node echoes; clinical case report and canine studies, Am. J. Cardiol. **31**:220, 1973.

57. Han, J., Malozzi, A. N., and Moe, G. K.: Sino-atrial reciprocation in the isolated rabbit heart, Circ. Res. **22**:355, 1968.

58. Paulay, K. L., Varghese, P. J., and Damato, A. N.: Sinus node reentry; an in vivo demonstration in the dog, Circ. Res. **32**:455, 1973.

59. Rytand, D. A.: The circus movement (entrapped circuit wave) hypothesis and atrial flutter, Ann. Intern. Med. **65**:125, 1966.

60. Wu, D., Amat-y-Leon, F., and others: Demonstration of sustained sinus and atrial re-entry as a mechanism of paroxysmal supraventricular tachycardia, Circulation **51**:234, 1976.

ABERRANCY OF JUNCTIONAL ESCAPE BEATS

61. Pick, A.: Aberrant ventricular conduction of escaped beats, Circulation **13**:702, 1956.

62. Sherf, L., and James, T. N.: The mechanism of aberration in late atrioventricular junctional beats, Am. J. Cardiol. **29**:529, 1972.

RETROGRADE P WAVE

63. Vitikainen, K. J., Waldo, A. L., and Hoffman, B. F.: Observations on the "retrograde" P wave, Circulation **45-46**(suppl. 2):104, 1972.

NONPAROXYSMAL JUNCTIONAL TACHYCARDIA

64. Kastor, J. A.: Digitalis intoxication in patients with atrial fibrillation, Circulation **47**:888, 1973.
65. Konecke, L. L., and Knoebel, S. B.: Nonparoxysmal junctional tachycardia complicating acute myocardial infarction, Circulation **45**:367, 1972.
66. Pick, A., and Dominquez, P.: Nonparoxysmal A-V nodal tachycardia complicating acute myocardial infarction, Circulation **16**:1022, 1957.
67. Rosen, K. M.: Junctional tachycardia: mechanisms, diagnosis, differential diagnosis and management, Circulation **47**:654, 1973.

VENTRICULAR TACHYCARDIA

68. El-Sherif, N., and Samet, P.: Multiform ventricular ectopic rhythm; evidence for multiple parasystolic activity, Circulation **51**:492, 1975.
69. Pick, A.: The electrophysiologic basis of parasystole and its variants. In Wellens, H. J. J., Lie, K. I., and Janse, M. J., editors: The conduction system of the heart: structure, function, and clinical implications, Philadelphia, 1976, Lea & Febiger.
70. Scherlag, B. J., Lazzara, R., Abelleira, J. L., and Samet, P.: Mechanisms of early and late arrhythmias due to myocardial ischemia and infarction (abstract), Circulation **46**(suppl. 2):59, 1972.
71. Wellens, H. J. J., Lie, K. I., and Durrer, D.: Further observations on ventricular tachycardia as studied by electrical stimulation of the heart; chronic recurrent ventricular tachycardia and ventricular tachycardia during acute myocardial infarction, Circulation **49**:647, 1974.

HEART BLOCK

72. Barold, S. S., and Friedberg, H. D.: Second degree atrioventricular block, Am. J. Cardiol. **33**:311, 1974.
73. Dhingra, R. C., and others: The significance of second degree atrioventricular block and bundle branch block, Circulation **44**:638, 1974.
74. El-Sherif, N., and Lazzara, R.: Evolution of second degree atrioventricular block in the His-Purkinje system following acute myocardial infarction (abstract), Circulation **54** (suppl. 2):191, 1976.

75. El-Sherif, N., Scherlag, B. J., and Lazzara, R.: Pathophysiology of second degree atrioventricular block; a unified hypothesis, Am. J. Cardiol. **35**:421, 1975.

BUNDLE BRANCH BLOCK AND HEMIBLOCK

76. Aranda, J. M., Befeler, B., Castellanos, A., and El-Sherif, N.: His bundle recordings; their contribution to the understanding of human electrophysiology, Heart Lung **5**:907, 1976.
77. Damato, A. N., and Lau, S. H.: Clinical value of the electrocardiogram of the conducting system, Prog. Cardiovasc. Dis. **13**:119, 1970.
78. Dhingra, R. C., Denes, P., Wu, D., Chuquimia, R., and Rosen, K. M.: Significance of second degree atrioventricular block and bundle branch block; observations regarding site and type of block, Circulation **44**:638, 1974.
79. Levites, R., and Haft, J.: Significance of first-degree heart block (prolonged P-R interval) in bifascicular block, Am. J. Cardiol. **34**:259, 1974.
80. Lichstein, E., Gupta, P. K., Chadda, K. D., and others: Findings of prognostic value in patients with incomplete bilateral bundle branch block complicating acute myocardial infarction, Am. J. Cardiol. **32**:913, 1974.
81. Lie, K. I., Wellens, H. J. J., Schuilenberg, R. M., and others: Factors influencing prognosis of bundle branch block complicating acute antero-septal infarction; the value of His bundle recordings, Circulation **50**:935, 1974.

WOLFF-PARKINSON-WHITE SYNDROME

82. Durrer, D., Schoo, L., and others: The role of premature beats in the initiation and termination of supraventricular tachycardia in the Wolff-Parkinson-White syndrome, Circulation **36**:644, 1967.
83. Gallagher, J. J., Sealy, W. C., Wallace, A. G., and Kasell, J.: Correlation between catheter electrophysiological studies and findings on mapping of ventricular excitation in the W. P. W. syndrome. In Wellens, H. J. J., Lie, K. I., and Janse, M. J., editors: The conduction system of the heart: structure, function, and clinical implications, Philadelphia, 1976, Lea & Febiger.
84. Wellens, H. J. J.: The electrophysiologic properties of the accessory pathway in the Wolff-Parkinson-White syndrome, In Wellens, H. J. J., Lie, K. I., and Janse, M. J., editors. The conduction system of the heart; structure, function, and clinical implications, Philadelphia, 1976, Lea & Febiger.

INDEX

Page numbers in boldface type indicate major discussion of the term.